GALEN. SELECTED BIBLIOGRAPHY (1965-2012)

Alberto J. Quiroga Puertas

Mª. Carmen García Sola

Bibliographic information published by the Deutsche Nationalbibliothek

The Deutsche Nationalbibliothek lists this publication in the Deutsche Nationalbibliografie; detailed bibliographic data are available in the Internet at http://dnb.d-nb.de .

ISBN 978-3-8325-3455-4

Logos Verlag Berlin GmbH
Comeniushof, Gubener Str. 47,
10243 Berlin
Tel.: +49 (0)30 42 85 10 90
Fax: +49 (0)30 42 85 10 92
INTERNET: http://www.logos-verlag.de

Foreword*

In a period in which the disciplines of the humanities are threatened by financial circumstances and the many wrong decisions made by the cultural elites, the figure of Galen of Pergamum stands out as a paradigmatic example of the importance to society of learned-men with boundless intellectual interests. He was a physician, a doctor, a surgeon, a writer, a philosopher, a polymath, a pepaideumenos. The depth of his paideia allowed him to regard human beings comprehensively and to deal with their bodies and souls. His importance in the cultural milieu of the second century A.D. has been accurately surveyed by Véronique Boudon-Millot in a recent biography (*Galien de Pergame. Un médecin grec à Rome*: Paris, 2012). Yet it is not his importance to his own times that has gained for him such a prominent place in the history of culture and of ideas but the continued relevance of his theories and principles throughout history and within different civilizations. Eastern cultures adopted and incorporated his legacy into their own philosophical, cultural and medical landscapes, and his influence remained a constant presence in the education of key figures (Alcuin of York, Agnellus of Ravenna, Burgundio of Pisa) in the constitution of medieval and Renaissance culture. Today, Galen's theories and writings are a fertile ground for several fields of knowledge, including ancient history, medicine and philosophy. Contrasting modern medical theories with Galen's or approaching his works from new intellectual or historiographical tendencies constitute the core of the current Galenic bibliographical production.

With this in mind, it is obvious that any effort to compose a complete bibliographical catalogue of Galenic studies is destined to fail. Indexes to scholarly works and bibliographical tools (e.g., L'Année Philologique, PubMed) in fields such as science, history or classical studies reveal new entries every day. Compiling, cataloguing and indexing this ever-increasing bibliographical production would therefore entail the production of a work destined to be outdated from its inception. Instead, our work aims to present a selection of the most representative and influential works on Galen from 1965 to 2012. By including bibliographical entries from disciplines as varied as neurology, ophthalmology, history of art, classics, codicology, etc., we aim to emphasize the multidisciplinary reception of Galen's work. In this sense, this bibliographical catalogue is different from Fichtner's

* We would like to acknowledge our gratitude to the Ancient Greek Department of the University of Granada, and to the research project directed by Prof. Juan Antonio López Férez "Obras de Galeno: medicina, otras ciencias, literatura, pensamiento" (FFI2010-22159).

seminal work (*Corpus Galenicum. Bibliographie der galenischen und pseudogalenischen Werke*) in that we mean to underline the great variety of fields in which Galen's influence is still felt –most notably among classicists.

The first part of the book ("Editions and Translations") is a list of works that shows that translating Galen's texts into modern languages -either because of the discovery of new texts or because textual emendations are needed- is unavoidable if our knowledge of his thought and theories is to be improved. "Main Websites" includes a brief list of webpages that contain references to the history of medicine and to sites dedicated to the presence of Galen on the internet. "Articles, papers, monographs, and volumes" is the longest section of the book, fulfilling its principle aim, which is to offer a general overview of the impact and influence of Galen's legacy in a plethora of fields of knowledge. His art was not restricted to medicine but comprised many areas that continue to be explored today, as the bibliographical references of this part of our catalogue prove. Thus, we hope that this work contributes to illustrating and emphasizing the ever-present influence of Galen in our culture.

EDITIONS AND TRANSLATIONS

2012

VAGELPOHL, U., "Galen, *Epidemics*, Book one: text, transmission, translation", in P.E. PORMANN (ed.), *Epidemics in Context: Hippocrates, Galen and Hunayn between East and West*, pp. 125-150, Berlin.

2011

ANDRÁS, L., "Galen on medicine. Excerpt from the "Introduction, or the physician"", *Orv Hetil* 152.4, pp. 142-145.

COOPER, G.M., *Galen, De diebus decretoriis, from Greek into Arabic: a critical edition, with translation and commentary, of Hunayn ibn Ishaq, Kitab Ayyam al-Buhran*. Farnham.

GARCÍA NOVO, E., *Galen. On the anomalous dyskrasia (De Inaequali intemperie)*. Berlin.

JOHNSTON, I. and HORSLEY, G.H.R., *Method of medicine*. London-Cambridge Mass.

NUTTON, V. and BOS, G., *Galen: on problematical movements*. Cambridge.

STEFANI, C., *De differentiis frebrium libri duo arabice conversi*. Pisa.

2010

BOUDON-MILLOT, V.; JOUANNA, J. and PIETROBELLI, A., *Galien. Tome IV, Ne pas se chagriner*. Paris.

GARCÍA SOLA, Mª.C., *Sobre los tipos; Contra los que escribieron los tipos, o El libro de los períodos; Sobre los días críticos*. Madrid.

LÓPEZ SALVÁ, M., *Del uso de las partes*. Madrid.

PINO CAMPOS, L.M., *Sobre la diferencia de los pulsos*. Madrid.

RUBIO FERNAZ, S., *Comentario al pronóstico de Hipócrates*. Madrid.

2009

BOULOGNE, J., *Méthode Thérapeutique*. Paris.

BRAIN, P., *Galen on bloodletting: a study of the origins, development, and validity of his opinions*. Cambridge.

GUNDERT, B., *Über die Verschiedenheit der Symptome*. Berlin.

LORUSSO, V., "Cinque nuovi frammenti di Galeno: edizione critica, traduzione, commento", *Galenos* 3, pp. 45-66.

ROSA P., *De Motu musculorum. Galenus*. Pisa-Roma.

2008

GARCÍA SOLA, Mª.C., "De Galeno *Que el mejor médico es filósofo*", in A. Pociña Pérez and J.Mª. García González (eds.), *En Grecia y Roma, II. Lecturas pendientes*, pp. 87-104, Granada.

GAROFALO, I., *L'anatomie des nerfs; L'anatomie des veines et des artères*. Paris.

INWOOD, B. and GERSON, L.P., *The Stoics Reader: selected writings and testimonia*. Indianapolis.

2007

BOUDON-MILLOT, V., *Tome I –Galien (Sur l'ordre de ses propres livres; Sur ses propres livres; Que l'excellent médecin est aussi philosophe)*. Paris.

— "Un traité perdu de Galien miraculeusement retrouvé, le *Sur l'inutilité de se chagriner*: texte grec et traduction française", in V. BOUDON-MILLOT; A. GUARDASOLE and C. MAGDELAINE (eds.), *La science médicale antique. Nouveaux regards*, pp. 72-123, Paris.

MANETTI, D., "Galeno, *De compositione medicamentorum per genera*, i 5, 7-8; ii 1, 2, 7, 8: vii 3, 5, 7, 9, 10, 11, 12 (pant 186)", in V.V.A.A, *Corpus dei papiri filosofici greci e latini I.2*, pp. 10-43, Florence.

SAKAI, T.; IKEDA, R., and SAWAI, T., "On bones for beginners", *Nihon Ishigaku Zasshi*. 53.3, pp. 353-421.

2006

FORTUNA, S. and RAIA, A., "*Corrigenda* and *addenda* to Diels' «*Galenica*» by Richard J. Durling. 3, Manuscripts and editions", *Traditio* 61, pp. 1-30.

JOHNSTON, I., *Galen. On diseases and symptoms*. Cambridge.

SAKAI, T.; IKEDA, R., and SAWAI, T., "On the anatomy of veins and arteries", *Nihon Ishigaku Zasshi* 52.2, pp. 211-272.

2005

BONED CÓLERA, P., "El texto dentro del texto: Filón, un poeta alejandrino en Galeno", in A. ALVAR EZQUERRA et al. (eds.), *Actas del XI congreso español de estudios clásicos*, pp. 253-260, Madrid.

BOUDON-MILLOT, V. and PIETROBELLI, A., "Galien ressucité: édition *princeps* du texte grec du *De propiis placitis*", *REG* 118.1, pp. 168-213.

GAROFALO, I. and DEBRU, A., *Galien. Les os pour les débutants; L'anatomie des muscles*. Paris.

NIETO IBÁÑEZ, J. Mª, *Trasíbulo o sobre si la salud depende de la medicina o de la gimnástica; Sobre el ejercicio con la pelotita; Sobre los placeres sexuales; Sobre el coma según Hipócrates; Sobre la diagnosis y curación de las afecciones del alma de cada uno*. Madrid.

PALMIERI, N. and GAROFALO, I., *Lectures galéniques: le «De pulsibus ad tirones» / Agnellus de Ravenne*. Saint-Étienne.

PINO CAMPOS, L.M., *Sinopsis de Galeno de su propia obra sobre pulsos*. Madrid.

SANTANA HENRÍQUEZ, G., *Sobre la composición de los medicamentos según los lugares. Libro II*. Las Palmas de Gran Canaria.

2004

ANDRÉS APARICIO, S., *Sobre la localización de las enfermedades (De locis affectis)*. Madrid.

DEMONT, P., "L'édition Vigoreus (1555) du traité hippocratique «*De humoribus*» et d'un «commentaire de Galien» à ce traité (= [Galien], «*De humoribus*», XIX, 485-496 Kühn), avec la traduction du «*De humoribus*» galénique ", in V. BOUDON-MILLOT and G. COBOLET (eds.), *Lire les médecins grecs à la Renaissance: aux origines de l'édition médicale*, pp. 43-59, Paris.

2003

BOULOGNE, J. and DELATTRE, D., *Systématisation de la médecine*. Paris.

FISCHER, K.-D., "*Galeni qui fertur ad Glauconem liber tertius ad fidem codicis Vindocinensis* 109", in I. GAROFALO and A. ROSELLI (ed.), *Galenismo e medicina tardoantica: fonti greche, latine e arabe*, pp. 287-354, Naples.

FORTUNA, S., "Histoire de la transmission et etablissement du texte du *De constitutione artis medicae*", in J. BOULOGNE and D. DELATTRE (eds.), *Galien. Systématisation de la médecine*, pp. 121-132, Lille.

POWELL, O., *On the properties of foodstuffs (De alimentorum facultatibus)*. Cambridge.

RODRÍGUEZ ALFAGEME, I., *Sobre las crisis*. Madrid.

SAKAI, T.; IKEDA, R. and TSUKISAWA, M., "Galen "On the anatomy of nerves"", *Nihon Ishigaku Zasshi* 16.2, pp. 105-107.

ZARAGOZA GRAS, J., *Sobre las facultades naturales: las facultades del alma siguen los temperamentos del cuerpo*. Madrid.

2002

BOUDON-MILLOT, V., *Galien: Introduction générale; Sur l'ordre de ses propres livres; Sur ses propres livres; Que l'excellent médecin devienne philosophe*. Paris.

GAROFALO, I., *Procedimenti anatomici*. Milan.

IHM, S., *Clavis commentariorum der antiken medizinischen Texte*. Leiden.

LÓPEZ SALVÁ, M., *Procedimientos anatómicos. Libros I-IX*. Madrid.

MARTÍNEZ MANZANO, T., *Tratados filosóficos y autobiográficos*. Madrid.

MEWALDT, I.; HELMREICH, G. and WESTENBERGER, I., *In Hippocratis de Natura hominis; In Hippocratis de victu acutorum; De diaeta Hippocratis in morbis acutis*. Karlshuld.

2001

ANASTASSIOU, A. and ANARGYROS, D.I., *Testimonien zum Corpus Hippocraticum. 2, Galen. 2, Hippokrateszitate in den übrigen Werken Galens einschliesslich der alten Pseudo-Galenica*. Göttingen.

BAZOU, A., *Galien. Que les facultés de l'âme suivent les tempéraments du corps*. Lille.

NICKEL, D., *Über die Ausformung der Keimlinge*. Berlin.

OTTE, C., *De plenitudine*. Wiesbaden.

SEZGIN, F., *The Alexandrian Compendium of Galen's work: Jawami' al-Iskandaraniyyin / translated by Hunayn ibn Ishâq*. Frankfurt.

2000

AL-DUBAYAN, A. M., *Galen, «Über die Anatomie der Nerven»: Originalschrift und alexandrinisches Kompendium in arabischer Überlieferung*. Berlin.

AMBJÖRN, L., *Qusta ibn Luqa on numbness: a book on numbness, its kinds, causes and treatment according to the opinion of Galen and Hippocrates*. Stockholm.

BOUDON-MILLOT, V., *Exhortation à l'étude de la médicine*. Paris.

— *Art medical*. Paris.

GAROFALO, I., *Anatomicarum administrationum libri qui supersunt nouem, earundem interpretatio Arabica Hunaino Isaaci filio ascripta. Libros V-IX continens*. Naples.

GRANT, M., *Galen on food and diet*. London.

PETIT, C., *Galien. Tome III: Le médecin*. Paris.

1999

COOPER, G.M., *Galen's «On critical days»: Greek medicine in Arabic*. Farnham.

DENOZ, L., *Transmission de l'art médical de la Grèce à l'Islam: étude du traité Sur les foetus de sept mois de Galien, de sa traduction par Hunayn b. Ishâq et de son commentaire par Tâbit b. Qurra*. Leuven.

MAGNALDI, G., *Claudii Galeni Pergameni Περὶ ψυχῆς παθῶν καὶ ἁμαρτημάτων*. Rome.

NUTTON, V., *On my own opinions*. Berlin.

1998

BARRAS, V.; BIRCHLER, T. and MORAND, A.F., *De la bile noire*. Paris.

DICKSON, K., *Stephanus the Philosopher and Physician. Commentary on Galen's Therapeutics to Glaucon*. Leiden.

HANKINSON, R.J., *Galen on antecedent causes*. Cambridge.

PELLEGRIN, P., *Traités philosophiques et logiques*. Paris.

1997

ANASTASSIOU, A. and IRMER, D., *Testimonien zum Corpus Hippocraticum. Teil II, Galen. 1. Band, Hippokrateszitate inden Kommentaren und im Glossar*. Göttingen.

ANDRÉS APARICIO, S., *Sobre la localización de las enfermedades*. Madrid.

FORTUNA, S., *Galeno, a Patrofilo sulla costituzione della medicina*. Berlin.

GARCÍA SOLA, Mª.C., *Sobre los lugares afectados*. Madrid.

LARA NAVA, D., *Sobre las facultades naturales: A Patrófilo; Sobre la constitución del arte médica*. Madrid.

SIMON, M., *Anatomie des Galen: sieben Bücher: zum ersten Male veröffentlicht nach den Handschriften einer arabischen Übersetzung des 9. Jahrh. n. Chr (Ἀνατομικῶν ἐγχειρήσεων βιβλίων 9-15)*. Osnabrück.

SINGER, P.N., *Galen Selected works*. Oxford.

TASSINARI, P., *De temperamentis*, Rome.

1996

DE LACY, Ph., *On the elements according to Hippocrates (De elementis ex Hippocratis)*. Berlin.

MORTARINO, M., *Sulle facoltà naturali*. Milan.

SMITH, E.S., *Galen on nerves, veins and arteries: a critical edition and translation from the Arabic, with notes, glossary and an introductory essay*. Ann Arbor.

1995

BARRAS, V.; TERPSICHORE, B. and MORAND, A.-F., *L'âme et ses passions: les passions et les erreurs de l'âme: les facultés de l'âme suivent les tempéraments du corps*. Paris.

1994

MUSITELLI, S., "Manuscript G. 108 inf. in the *Ambrosiana* library in Milan", *Hist Sci Med.* 28.3, pp. 249-254.

1993

DEAN-JONES, D.E., *On the constitution of the art of medicine*. Austin.

1992

BARZEL, U.S., *Maimonides' medical writings. The Art of Cure: extracts from Galen*. Haifa.

DE LACY, Ph., *On semen*. Berlin.

DURLING, R.J., *Galenus Latinus, II : Burgundio of Pisa's translation of Galen's Περὶ τῶν πεπονθότων τόπων, De interioribus*. Stuttgart.

LARRAIN, C., *Galens Kommentar zu Platons Timaios*. Stuttgart.

TIELEMAN. T., *Galen and Chrysippus: argument and refutation in the De Placitis, Books II-III*. Utrecht.

1991

BARIGAZZI, A., *Galeno. Sull' ottima maniera d'insegnare. Esortazione alla medicina*. Berlin.

GAROFALO, I., *Galeno, Procedimenti anatomici*. Milan.

HANKINSON, R., *Galen. On the therapeutic method: books I-II*. Oxford.

1990

SZARMACH, M., "*Adhortatio ad artes addiscendas*", *Meander* 45, pp. 209-223.

1989

PALMIERI, N., *L'antica versione latina del De sectis di Galeno: (Pal. lat. 1090)*. Pisa.

1988

ISKANDAR, Z., *De optimo medico cognoscendo*. Berlin.

1987

IERACI BIO, A.M., *De bonis malisque sucis, testo*. Naples.

1986

ATZPODIEN, J., *Galens Subfiguratio empirica. Deutsche Übersetzung und inhatliche Erlaüterungen der medizintheoretischen Ansätze bei den griechischen Empirikern*. Husum.

BALDASSARRI, M., *Galeno. Dalla Introduzione alla dialectica*. Como.

GALLI CALDERINI, I.J., *Galeno. Nobilità delle arti (Protepticus)*. Naples.

GAROFALO, I., *Anatomicarum administrationum libri qui supersunt novem. Earundem interpretatio Arabico Hunaino Isaaci filio abscripta. Tomus prior libros I-IV continens*. Napoli.

OCHOA, J.A. and SANZ MINGOTE, L., *Galeno: Exhortación al aprendizaje de las artes. Sobre la mejor doctrina. El mejor médico es también filósofo. Sobre las escuelas, a los que se inician*. Madrid.

1985

GARCÍA BALLESTER, L.; SÁNCHEZ SALOR, E., and DURLING, R. J., *Arnaldo Villanova Opera medica omnia XV: Commentum supra tractatum Galieni de malicia complexionis diverse, Doctrina Galieni de interioribus*. Barcelona.

GOSS, C.M. and CHODKOWSKI, E.G., “Whether blood is contained in the arteries of the living animal by Galen of Pergamon: a translation”, *Anat.Rec*, 213, pp. 1-6.

— ““‘On Bones for Beginners” by Galen of Pergamon: a translation with commentary”, *Am.J.Anat* 169, pp. 59-74.

GREPPIN, J.A.C., *Bark' Galianosi. The Greek-Armenian dictionary to Galen*. New York.

LEVET, J.P., “L'*Institutio logica* di Galeno. La syllogistique, traduction acompagnée de notes”, in V.V.A.A., *D'Hippocrate à Alcuin*, pp. 57-80, Limoges.

WALZER, R. and FREDE, M., *Galen. Three Treatises on the nature of science. On the sects for beginners, An outline of empiricism, On medical experience*. Indianapolis.

1984

DE LACY, Ph., *De placitis Hippocratis et Platonis*. Berlin.

FURLEY, D.J. and WILKIE, J.S., *Galen, On respiration and arteries*. New York.

MENGHI, M. and VEGETTI, M., *Le passioni e gli errore dell'anima*. Venice.

1983

FICHTNER, G., *Corpus Galenicum. Verzlichnis der galenischen und pseudogalenischen Schriften*. Tübingen.

1982

OTERO, M. and RAMIREZ TREJO, A., *Iniciación a la dialéctica*. Mexico.

PRITCHER, C.D., *Ioahannis Alexandrini Commentaria in librum De sectis Galeni*. Leiden.

V.V.A.A., *Agnellus of Ravenna. Lectures on Galen's De sectis*. New York.

WASSERSTEIN, A., *Galen's commentary on the Hippocratic treatise Airs, waters, places in the Hebrew translation of Salomon ha-Me'ati*. Jerusalem.

1980

DE LACY, Ph., *De placitis Hippocratis et Platonis* VI-IX. Berlin.

1979

KOLLESCH, J. and NICKEL, D., *Antike Heilkunst. Ausgewählte Texte aus dem medizinischen Schrifttum der Griechen und Römer*. Leipzig.

NUTTON, V., *De praecognitione. On prognosis*. Berlin.

SIDER, D. and McVAUGH, M., "Galen on Tremor, Palpitation, Spasm and Rigor", *Trans. Stud. Coll. Phys. Philadelphia* 1.3, pp. 183-210.

1978

DE LACY, Ph., *De placitis Hippocratis et Platonis, Libri I-V*. Berlin.

GAROFALO, I. and VEGETTI, M., *Opere scelte di Galeno*. Torino.

MITROPOULOS, K., *Glossarion Hippokrátous idíai katà Erotianón kaì Galenón*. Athens.

PETERS, H., *Über die Heilkunst*. Hamburg.

1977

EDLOW, R.B., *Galen on language and ambiguity. A translation of Galen's De captionibus (On fallacies)*. Leiden.

1976

DURLING, R.J., *Galenus Latinus, I. Burgundio of Pisa's translation of Galen's Περὶ κράσεων, "De complexionibus"*. Berlin.

GIUSTA, M., *Quod qualitates incorporeae sint*. Torino.

NUTTON, V., *Karl-Gottlob Kühn and his edition of the works of Galen*. Oxford.

SIEGEL, R.E., *On the affected parts*. Basel.

USOBIAGA, B., "El mejor médico también es filósofo", *BIEH* 10, pp. 133-151.

1974

ZORGNIOTTI, A.W., "Galenic urology. Translation of urologic portions of *De Locis Affectis* (Book I, Chapter 1)", *Urology* 8, pp. 638-642.

1973

BIESTERFELDT, T.H., *Dass die Kräfte der Seele den Mischungen des Körpers folgen*. Wiesbaden.

EBBESEN, S., "*Galeni libellus de captionibus*. New Manuscripts", *Hermes* 101, pp. 374-379.

MARINONE, N., *La dieta dimagrante*. Torino.

PENELLA, R.J. and HALL, Th.S., "Galen on the best constitution of our body: Introduction, translation and notes", *BHM* 47, pp. 282-296.

1972

ABBALLE, M. and PAZZINI, A., *I classici medicina dell' età greco-romana III: Galeno, Il commentario al trattato Delle articolazioni*. Rome.

ANDREONI, E., *I tre commentari al trattato delle fratture di Ippocrate*. Rome.

DEMUTH, G., *Ps.-Galeni De dignotione ex insomnis. Ausgabe mit Übersetzung und Kommentar*. Gottingen.

EDLOW, R.B., *Galen's On ambiguity. An English translation of Galen's De captionibus*. Philadelphia.

FABRICIUS, C., *Galens Excerpte aus alteren Pharmakologen*. Berlin.

1971

BECCARIA, A., "Sulle tracce di un antico canone latino di Ippocrate e di Galeno, III: Quattro opere di Galeni nei commenti della scuola di Ravenna all'inizio del medioevo", *IMU* 14, pp. 1-23.

NICKEL, D., *Über die Anatomie der Gebärmutter*. Berlin.

THEOHARIDES, T.C., "Galen on Marasmus", *JHM* 26, pp. 369-390.

1970

KOTRC, R.F., *Galen's On phlebotomy against the Erasistrateans at Rome (Galeni De venae sectione adversus Erasistrateos Romae degentes).* Washington.

STROHMAIER, G., *Galen's Buch über die Verchiedenheit der homoiomeren Körperteil.* Berlin.

STROPPIANA, L., "Il trattato di Galeno su la sezione degli organi che articolano i suoni (traduzione e commento)", *Riv.Stor.Med* 14, pp. 131-148.

1969

MOORE, M.G., *Galen. Introduction to the bones. A critical edition whith translation and indices*. Michigan.

SMITH, E.S., *Galen on nerves, veins and arteries. A critical edition and translation from the Arabic, with notes, glossary and introductory essay.* Wisconsin.

WASZINK, J.H., *Galeni Exhortatio ad bonas artes praesertim medicinam. De optimo docendi genere, et Qualem oporteat esse medicum, Erasmo interprete*. Amsterdam.

1968

ALEXANDERSON, B., *Testkritischer Kommentar Hippokratischen Prognostikon und Bemerkungen zu Galens Prognostikonkommentar*. Stockholm.

LYONS, M., *On the parts of medicine. On cohesive causes. On regimen in acute diseases in accordance with the theories of Hippocrates.* Berlin.

MAY, M.T., *On the usefulness of the parts of the body* I-II. New York.

PERAZZI, F., "Il glossario Ippocratico di Galeno (traduzione del proemio, commento e considerazioni)", *Riv.Stor.Med.* 12, pp. 28-44.

REEDY, J., *De tumoribus praeter naturam.* Michigan.

RUSCH, F.A., *Galen's De placitis Hippocratis et Platonis, L. VIII, A Text and commentary.* Northwestern.

SACINO, G., "Il libro "*De catharticis*" attribuito a Galeno. (Traduzione e commento)", *Riv.Stor.Med* 12, pp. 217-229.

1967

BUERGEL, J. Ch., *Averroes contra Galenum. Das Kapitel von der Atmung im Colliget des Averroes als ein Zeugnis mittelalterlich-islamischer Kritik an Galen.* Göttingen.

1966

BACHMANN, P., *Abhandlung darüber, dass der vorzügliche Artz Philosoph sein muss (Quod optimus medicus sit quoque philosophus)*. Göttingen.

RESCHR, N., *Galen and the syllogism. An examination of the thesis that Galen originated the 4th figure of the syllogism in the ligth of new data from Arabic sources, incluiding an Arabic text edition and annotaded translation of Ibn al-Salah's treatise: On the 4th figure of the categorical syllogism*. Pittsburg.

1965

KIEFFER, J.S., *Institutio logica*. Oxford.

MALATO, M.T., *Giambattista Morgagni (1682-1771)*. Rome.

RESCHER, N. and MARMURA, M.E., *The refutation by Alexander of Aphrodisias Galen's treatise On the theory of motion*. Islamabad.

RIESE, W. and HARKINS, P.W., *Galen's On the passions and errors of the soul*. Ohio.

MAIN WEBSITES

HISTORY OF MEDICINE:

http://www.ucl.ac.uk/~ucgajpd/medicina%20antiqua/index.html

http://www.orient-mediterranee.com/spip.php?rubrique314&lang=fre

https://www.hsl.virginia.edu/historical/artifacts/antiqua/galen.cfm

http://www.nchm.ac.uk/

http://www.hsls.pitt.edu/histmed

GALEN ON THE INTERNET:

http://robl.de/galen/galen.htm

http://www.biusante.parisdescartes.fr/histmed/medica/galien_vf.htm

http://www.cndp.fr/archive-musagora/jeux/jeuxfr/galien.htm

http://www.medarus.org/Medecins/MedecinsTextes/galien_claude.html

http://www.iep.utm.edu/galen/

BIBLIOGRAPHICAL CATALOGUES:

http://galen.bbaw.de/online-publications/hippokrates-und-galenbibliographie-fichtner

http://cmg.bbaw.de/epubl/online/editionencmg_05.html

http://cmg.bbaw.de/online-publikationen/Galen-Bibliographie_2012_08_28.pdf

http://www.nndb.com/people/788/000087527/bibliography/

http://www.idref.fr/02776897X

http://www2.biusante.parisdescartes.fr/hm/?refbiogr=6514

ARTICLES, PAPERS, MONOGRAPHS AND VOLUMES

2012

ALESSI, R., "The Arabic version of Galen's Commentary on Hippocrates' *Epidemics*, Book Two, as a source for the Hippocratic Text: First Remarks", in P.E. PORMANN (ed.), *Epidemics in Context: Hippocrates, Galen and Hunayn Between East and West*, pp. 71-90, Berlin.

BECCHI, F., "The doctrine of the passions: Plutach, Posidonius and Galen", in L.R. LANZILLOTTA and I. MUÑOZ GALLARTE (eds.), *Plutarch in the Religious and Philosophical Discourse of Late Antiquity*, pp. 43-54, Leiden.

BOUDON-MILLOT, V., *Galien de Pergame. Un médecin grec à Rome*. Paris.

CERNY, K, "Early modern "citation index"? Medical authorities in academic treatises on plague (1480-1725)", *Prague Med Rep*. 113.2, pp. 119-135.

CHIPMAN, L., "Recipes by Hippocrates, Galen and Hunayn in the *Epidemics* and in Medieval Arabic Pharmacopoeias", in P.E. PORMANN (ed.), *Epidemics in Context: Hippocrates, Galen and Hunayn Between East and West*, pp. 285-302, Berlin.

EIJK, P.J., "Exegesis, explanation and Epistemology in Galen's *Commentaries on Epidemics*, Books One and Two", in P. PORMANN (ed.), *Epidemics in Context: Greek commentaries on Hippocrates in the Arabic tradition*, pp. 25-48, Berlin.

FICHTNER, G., *Corpus Galenicum. Bibliographie der galenischen und pseudogalenischen Werke*. Berlin.

GOUREVITCH, D., "The doctor and the consul. Relations between Galen and Flavius Boethos under Marcus Aurelius", *Hist Sci Med*. 46.1, pp. 55-65.

HALLUM, B., "A New Manuscript: Istanbul, Süleymaniye Kütüphanesi, MS Ayasofya 3592", in P. PORMANN (ed.), *Epidemics in Context: Greek commentaries on Hippocrates in the Arabic tradition*, pp. 15-22, Berlin.

—"The Arabic Reception of Galen's Commentary on Hippocrates' *Epidemics*", in P.E. PORMANN (ed.), *Epidemics in Context: Hippocrates, Galen and Hunayn Between East and West*, pp. 185-210, Berlin.

HARRISON A.P.; HANSEN S.H. and BARTELS E.M., "Transdermal Opioid Patches for Pain Treatment in Ancient Greece", *Pain Pract*. 12.8, pp. 620-625.

HIRAI, H., "Formative power, soul and intellect in Nicolò Leoniceno between the arabo-latin tradition and the Renaissance of the Greek commentators", in P. BAKKER et al. (eds.), *Psychology and other disciplines: a Case of Cross-Disciplinary Interaction*, pp. 297-324, Boston-Leiden.

HOLMES, B. "Sympathy between Hippocrates and Galen: The Case of Galen's Commentary on Epidemics II", in P.E. PORMANN (ed.), *Epidemics in Context: Hippocrates, Galen and Hunayn Between East and West*, pp. 49-71, Berlin.

JIMÉNEZ, L., *Terapia floral evolutiva: la vía iniciática de E. Bach*. Malaga.

KING, H., “History without historians? Medical history and the internet”, *Social History of Medicine* 25, pp. 212-221

KOUTROUMPAS, D.C. and KOLETSI-KOUNARI, H., “Galen on dental anatomy and physiology”, *J Hist Dent*. 60.1, pp. 37-49.

MAZZUCCHI, C.M., “In Galenun novum”, *Aevum* 86.1, pp. 251-263.

NUTTON, V., “Galen and Roman medicine: or can a Greek become Latin?”, *European Review* 20.4, pp. 534-542.

RODWAY, G.W., “The foundations of wilderness medicine: some historical features”, *Wilderness Environ Med*. 23.2, pp. 165-169.

ROSELLI, A. “Vino profumato e pane appena sfornato, ovvero guarire e nutrire con gli odori: Ippocrate *Epidemie* VI 8.7 letto da Areteo, Galeno e Giovanni Alessandrino”, in A. CARANNANTE and M. d’ ACUNTO (eds.), *I profumi nelle società antiche: produzione, usi, valori simbolici*, pp. 265-276, Salerno.

SNYDER, G., “The Classroom in the text: Exegetical practices in Justin and Galen”, in S. PORTER and A. PITTS (eds.), *Christian Origins and Graeco-Roman Culture*, pp. 663-685, Leiden.

STROHMAIER, G., “Galen the Pagan and Hunayn the Christian: Specific Transformations in the Commentaries on Airs, Waters, Places and Epidemics”, in P.E. PORMANN (ed.), *Epidemics in Context: Hippocrates, Galen and Hunayn Between East and West*, pp. 171-184, Berlin.

TOTELIN, L., “And to end on a poetic note: Galen’s authorial strategies in the pharmacological books’”, *Studies in History and Philosophy of Science* 43, pp. 307–315.

2011

AIRD, W.C., “Discovery of the cardiovascular system: from Galen to William Harvey”, *J Thromb Haemost*. 9.1, pp. 118-129.

BAZOU, A., *Γαληνού Ότι ταις του σώματος κράσεσιν αι της ψυχής δυνάμεις έπονται*. Athens.

BOUDON-MILLOT, V. “De Pythàgore a Maxime Planude en passant par Galien: la fortune excepcionnelle de l’adage médico-philosophique ὡς μήτε πεῖνην μήτε ῥιγοῦν μήτε διψῆν”, in L. PERILLI et al. (eds.), *Officina Hippocratica*, pp. 3-28, Berlin.

BROCKMANN, C., “Manuskriptanalyse und Edition II. Weitere Beispiele aus Galens Kommentar zu Hippokrates, *De articulis*”, en L. PERILLI et al. (eds.), *Officina Hippocratica*, pp. 329-343, Berlin.

BUJALKOVA, M., "Rufus of Ephesus and his contribution to the development of anatomical nomenclature", *Acta Med Hist Adriat.* 9.1, pp. 89-100.

CILLIERS, L., "The Didactic Letters Prefacing Marcellus' *On Drugs* as Evidence for the Expertise and Reputation of Doctors in the Late Roman Empire", in M. HORSTMANSHOFF (ed.), *Hippocrates and medical education*, pp. 401-418, Leuven.

COOPER, G.M., "Galen and astrology: a Mésalliance?", *Early Sci Med.* 16.2, pp. 120-146.

EIJK, P.J., "Modes and degrees of soul-body relationship in *On Regimen*", in L. PERILLI et al. (eds.), *Officina Hippocratica*, pp. 255-270, Berlin.

FISCHER, K.D., "*Ex occidente lux*: Greek medical works as represented in pre-Salernitan Latin translations", in L. PERILLI et al. (eds.), *Officina Hippocratica*, pp. 29-56, Berlin.

GAROFALO, I., "I lemmi ippocratici di *Epidemie* II e la traduzione araba del commento di Galeno", in L. PERILLI et al. (eds.), *Officina Hippocratica*, pp. 57-76, Berlin.

— "Gli estratti di 'Ali ibn Ridwan dal commento di Galeno agli *umori* di Ippocrate", *Galenos* 5, pp. 113-172.

GOUREVITCH, D., *Pour une archéologie de la médicine romaine*. Paris.

HAVRDA, M., "Galenus Christianus? The Doctrine of Demonstration in *Stromata* VIII and the Question of its Source", *VCh* 65.4, pp. 343-375.

KING, H., "Galen and the widow. Towards a history of therapeutic masturbation in ancient gynaecology'", *Eugesta* 1, pp. 205-235.

KOUSOULIS, A.; ATHANASOPOULOU, I. and POULAKOU REBELAKOU, E., "How to cope with disaster loss and mourning: Galen's paper which was lost for centuries", *Vesalius* 17.2, pp. 99-101.

LAFONT, O., *Galien glorifié, Galien contesté*. Paris.

LAMI, A., "Una *distinctio* azzardata e la dottrina delle sei virtù dell' anima in Galeno", in L. PERILLI al. (eds.), *Officina Hippocratica*, pp. 117-126, Berlin.

LÓPEZ PÉREZ, M., "Autoritarismo, persuasión y didáctica de la medicina en la obra de Galeno", in G. BRAVO CASTAÑEDA and R. GONZÁLEZ SALINERO (eds.), *Propaganda y persuasión en el mundo romano*, pp. 413-422, Madrid.

MARERI, L., "Galeno, *De ordine librorum suorum:* letture da una nuova collazione dei mss. *Ambr. gr.* 659 e *vlatadon*", *Galenos* 5, pp. 173-174.

MATTERN, S., "Galen and his patients", *Lancet* 378, pp. 478-479.

MOREAU, E., "The Galenic content of Isaac Beeckman's medical ideas (1617-1629)", *Studium* 4.3, pp. 137-151.

NICHOLLS, M.C., "Galen and libraries in the *Peri Alupias*", *JRS* 101, pp. 123-142.

PAPAVRAMIDOU, N.; THOMAIDIS, V. and FISKA, A., "The ancient surgical bloodletting method of arteriotomy", *J Vasc Surg*. 54.6, pp. 1842-1844.

PERILLI, L., "Nuovi manoscritti del Glossario Ippocratico di Galeno e considerazioni stemmatiche. *Codex olim Mosquensis, Codex Bodleianus Holkhamensis 92*", in L. PERILLI et al. (eds.), *Officina Hippocratica*, pp. 177-202, Berlin.

PERILLI, L. et al. (eds.), *Officina Hippocratica*. Berlin.

PORMANN, P.E., "The formation of the Arabic pharmacology between tradition and innovation", *Ann Sci*. 68.4, pp. 493-515.

RETIEF, F.P. and CILLIERS, L., "Breast cancer in antiquity", *Afr Med J.* 101.8, pp. 513-515.

ROSELLI, A., "I maestri di Galeno, Galeno come maestro", in A. ROSELLI and R. VELARDI (eds.), *L'insegnamento delle Technai nelle culture antiche*, pp. 53-70, Pisa-Rome.

SIMON, F. and STEGER, F., "Bow legged adjectives in ancient literature", *Sudhoffs Arch.* 95.2, pp. 209-221

SOLOMON, J.A., "Galen disease: delusions of grandeur in an authoritative clinical investigator", *Arch Dermatol* 147.6, p. 723.

TOMMASO, R., "«Asini per uccelli»: una noterella al testo di *De indolentia*", *Galenos* 5, pp. 21-26.

V.V.A.A., "The scientific revolutions in medicine in XVII-XIX centuries: disclaimer of Galenism and initiation of natural-scientific foundations of medicine. Report 4. The disclaimer of Galen concepts on principles of structure and mechanisms of functioning of nervous system", *Probl Sotsialnoi Gig Zdravookhranenniiai Istor Med*. Mar-Apr (2), pp. 47-51.

2010

ANASTASSIOU, A., "Unbekannte hippokratische Aphorismen bei Theophilos Protospatharios' «*De urinis*»?", *RhM* 153.1, pp. 92-107.

ARATA, L., "Un caso di sterilità temporanea in *mul.* 19", *Galenos* 4, pp. 13-16.

BOUDON-MILLOT, V., "Galien de Pergame et la pratique épistolaire", in P. LAURENCE and F. GUILLAUMONT (eds.), *Les écritures de la douleur dans l'épistolair de l'Antiquité à nos jours*, pp. 113-132, Tours.

— "Aux origins de la thériaque: la recette d' Andromaque", *Revue d'Histoire de la Pharmacie* LVIII (nº 367), pp. 261-270.

CILLIERS, L., "The didactic letters prefacing Marcellus' on drugs as evidence for the expertise and reputation of doctors in the late Roman empire", in M. HORSTMANSHOFF (ed.), *Hippocrates and medical education*, pp. 401-418, Leiden.

ETZELMÜLLER, G. and WEISSENRIEDER, A. (eds.), *Religion und Krankheit*. Darmstadt.

EVERETT, N., "New evidence for the use of the latin suffix *-aster*. Contributions to tracing a linguistic phenomenon and the vestiges of lost ancient sources on pharmacy: the *Alphabetum Galieni*", *Galenos* 4, pp. 185-206.

FORTUNA, S., "Galeno e le traduzioni medievali: il «*De purgantium medicamentorum facultate*»", *MedSec* 22.1-3, pp. 297-341.

GARCÍA SOLA, Mª.C., "Galeno. La Odontoestomatología: avance y retroceso", *Florentia Iliberritana* 21, pp. 133-155.

GAROFALO, I., "I commenti a *Epidemie* III e VI", *Galenos* 4, pp. 229-256.

— "Postilla a I commenti a *Epidemie*", *Galenos* 4, pp. 257-258.

GÄRTNER, F., "Prolegomena zu einer edition von Galens schrift *De locis affectis*", *Galenos* 4, pp. 47-80.

GILL, C., *Naturalistic psychology in Galen and Stoicism*. Oxford.

HANKINSON, R. J., "Galen", in P.G. LLOYD (ed.), *The Cambridge History of Philosophy in Late Antiquity*, pp. 210-231, Cambridge.

HANSON, A.E., "Doctors' literacy and papyri of medical content", in M. HORSTMANSHOFF (ed.), *Hippocrates and medical education*, pp. 187-204, Leiden.

HOLMES, B., *The symptom and the subject: the emergence of the physical body in ancient Greece*. Princeton.

HORSTMANSHOFF, M. (ed.), *Hippocrates and medical education*. Leiden.

IERACI BIO, A.N., "Un *excerptum* del commento di Stefano all' *Ad glauconem* di Galeno (cap. 6) nel trivult. 685", *Galenos* 4, pp. 163-172.

JIRSA, F. and WINIWARTER, V., "Intestinal helminths in the works of Galen", *Wien Klin Wochenschr.* 122.3, pp. 14-18.

JOHNSON, W.A., *Readers and reading Culture in the High Roman Empire: a study of elite communities*. Oxford.

JOUANNA, J., "Hippocrates as Galen's teacher", in M. HORSTMANSHOFF (ed.), *Hippocrates and medical education*, pp. 1-21, Leiden.

LAES, C., "The Educated Midwife in the Roman Empire. An example of differential equations", in M. HORSTMANSHOFF (ed.), *Hippocrates and medical education*, pp. 261-286, Leiden.

LAMI, A., "Sul testo del *De propriis placitis* di Galeno", *Galenos* 4, pp. 81-126.

LÓPEZ FÉREZ, J.A., "Some Remarks by Galen about the Teaching and Studying of Medicine", in M. HORSTMANSHOFF (ed.), *Hippocrates and medical education*, pp. 361-400, Leiden.

LÓPEZ PÉREZ, M., *Ginecología y patología sexual femenina en las Colecciones Médicas de Oribasio*. Oxford.

LUCARINI, C.M., "Congetture al nuovo Galeno", *Philologus* 154.2, pp. 331-337.

MANETTI, D., "Problemi di tradizione tardoantica e medievale di Galeno *De compositione medicamentorul per genera"*, in V. BOUDON-MILLOT et al. (eds.), *VIe colloque international. Storia della tradizione e edizione dei medici greci*, pp. 129-142, Naples.

MARASCO, G., "The Curriculum of Studies in the Roman Empire and the Cultural Role of Physicians", in M. HORSTMANSHOFF (ed.), *Hippocrates and medical education*, pp. 205-220, Leiden.

MARGANNE, M.-H., "La «*Bibliothèque médicale*» de Photios", *MedSec* 22.1-3, pp. 509-530.

MARTELLI, M., "Medicina ed alchimia. '*Estratti galenici*' nel corpus degli scritti alchemici siriaci di Zosimo", *Galenos* 4, pp. 207-228.

MORELLI, F., "P. Ant. III 139 fr. 1: un frammento di Galeno, *De compositione medicamentorum per genera* VII 10 - e di P. Ant. III 186?", *ZPE* 172, pp. 203-207.

MUGNAI, D., "Nicolò Leoniceno interprete di Galeno sulla «*causa coniuncta*»", *MedSec* 22.1-3, pp. 593-610.

PAPAVRAMIDOU, N. and TZIAKAS, D., "Galen on syncope", *Int J Cardiol*. 142.3, pp. 242-244.

PETIT, C., "Hippocrates in the pseudo-Galenic Introduction: Or how was medicine taught in Roman times?", in M. HORSTMANSHOFF (ed.), *Hippocrates and medical education*, pp. 343-360, Leiden.

RAIOLA, T., "Alle origini di un falso galenico: il «*Commento*» al «*De alimento*» e una citazione di Sabino", *AION(filol)* 32, pp. 101-110.

RETSAS, S., "Galen's "errors"", *Lancet* 376, p. 686.

ROSA, P., "Contributi umanistici e rinascimentali al testo del *De motu musculorum* di Galeno", *Galenos* 4, pp. 259-262.

ROSELLI, A., "Libri e biblioteche a Roma al tempo di Galeno: la testimonianza del *De indolentia", Galenos* 4, pp. 127-148.

ROSEN, R., "Galen, satire and the compulsion to instruct", in M. HORSTMANSHOFF (ed.), *Hippocrates and medical education*, pp. 323-342, Leiden.

RUSSELL, G.A., "After Galen: Late Antiquity and the Islamic world", *Handb Clin Neurol.* 95, pp. 61-77.

SLUITER, I., "Textual Therapy. On The Relationship Between Medicine And Grammar in Galen", in M. HORSTMANSHOFF (ed.), *Hippocrates and medical education*, pp. 23-52, Leiden.

SMITH, C.U., "The triune brain in antiquity: Plato, Aristotle, Erasistratus", *Hist Neurosci.* 19.1, pp. 1-14.

STROHMAIER, G., "Galenismus zwischen Gottvertrauen und «prophetischer Medizin» im Islam", in G. ETZELMÜLLER and A. WEISSENRIEDER (eds.), *Religion und Krankheit*, pp. 97-106, Darmstadt.

TIELEMAN, T., "Religion and therapy in Galen", in G. ETZELMÜLLER, G. and A. WEISSENRIEDER (eds.), *Religion und Krankheit*, pp. 83-95, Darmstadt.

ZAGO, G., "La favola esopica delle due bisacce: restauri testuali e note esegetiche a Galeno, "De an. aff. dig. et cur." 2,7 a Ps.-Acrone, "schol. Hor. sat. 2,3299" e alla "Parafrasi Bodleiana" di Babrio", *MH* 67, pp. 7-17.

ZYLBERMAN. M, and YOUNG P., "Pericardial disease: from antiquity to the ultrasound", *Med Mex.* 146.5, pp. 348-353.

2009

ANDÒ, V., "Sogni erotici e seme femminile nella antica medicina greca", *MedSec* 21.2, pp. 663-691.

ARUTA, A.; MARENCO, M. and MARINOZZI, S., "Dalla suffusio al cristallino: storia della cataratta attraverso gli strumenti del Museo della Storia della Medicina della «*Sapienza*» Università di Roma", *MedSec* 21.1, pp. 403-428.

AYDIN, K. and QUINTERN, D., "Die verschlungenen Wege des Wissens", *AW* 40.5, pp. 35-39.

BAN, D., "The history of the study of *On ancient medicine*", *Uisahak.* 18.1, pp. 91-105.

BOUDON-MILLOT, V., "Galen's βίος and μέθοδος: from ways of life to path of knowledge", in C. GILL; T. WHITMARSH and J. WILKINS, (eds.), *Galen and the world of knowledge*, pp. 175-189, Cambridge.

— "Le *De dignotione ex insomniis* (Kühn VI, 832-835) est'il un traité authentique de Galien?", *REG* 122, pp. 617-634.

— "Anecdote et antidote: fonction du récit anecdotique dans le discours galénique sur la thériaque", in C. BROCKMANN; W. BRUNSCHÖN, and O.OVERWIEN (eds.), *Antike Medizin im Schnittpunkt von Geistes- und Naturwissenschaften*, pp. 45-61, Berlin-New York.

BROCKMANN, C., "Medizin und Körperdarstellung: zur Wiederentdeckung der antiken Chirurgie in der Renaissance", in D. GALL and A. WOLKENHAUER (eds.), *Laokoon in Literatur und Kunst*, pp. 146-159, Berlin.

— "«Gross war der Name Galens»: die Selbstdarstellung eines Arztes in seinen wissenschaftlichen Werken", *MHJ* 44.2, pp. 109-129.

BROCKMANN, C. and BRUNSCHÖN, C. (eds.), *Antike Medizin im Schnittpunkt von Geistes- und Naturwissenschaften*. Berlin.

CHIARADONNA, R., "Galen and Middle Platonism", in C. GILL; T. WHITMARSH and J. WILKINS, (eds.), *Galen and the world of knowledge*, pp. 243-260, Cambridge.

CIRANNI, R., "When Galen met Paracelsus: a paleodermatological case of luetic gumma care", *Arch Dermatol*. 145.1, p. 101.

DIAMANDOPOULOS, A. and GOUDAS, P., "Juxtaposition of Actuarius' versus Galen's ideas on renal physiology: the impact of 12 centuries", *J Nephrol.* 22.14, pp. 21-32.

EIJK, P.J., "«Aristotle! What a thing for you to say!»: Galen's engagement with Aristotle and Aristotelians", in C. GILL; T. WHITMARSH and J. WILKINS, (eds.), *Galen and the world of knowledge*, pp. 261-281, Cambridge.

FISCHER, K.-D., "Galen, Pardalas, and sundry delights for the student of ancient Greek medicine", *Galenos* 3, pp. 161-176.

FISCHER, K.-D. et al., "Congetture e emendamenti inediti sui testi medici", *Galenos* 3, pp. 181-191.

FLEMMING, R., "Demiurge and emperor in Galen's world of knowledge", in C. GILL; T. WHITMARSH and J. WILKINS, (eds.), *Galen and the world of knowledge*, pp. 59-84, Cambridge.

FORTUNA, S., "Galeno e le traduzioni latine", *Bollettino della facoltà di Medicina e Chirurgia dell'Università Politecnica delle Marche* 12, pp. 2-7.

FREDE, D. and BURKHARD, R. (eds.), *Body and soul in ancient philosophy*. Berlin.

FULLERTON, J.B. and SILVERMAN, M.E., "Claudius Galen of Pergamum: authority of medieval medicine", *Clin Cardiol*. 32.11, pp. 82-83.

GAROFALO, I., "Postilla all'articolo gli scoli al *De Sectis*", *Galenos* 3, pp. 67-68.

—"I commenti alle «*Epidemie*» e la loro traduzione araba", *Galenos* 3, pp. 113-160.

GAROFALO, I.; LAMI, A. and ROSELLI, A. (eds.), *Sulla tradizione indiretta dei testi medici greci*. Pisa.

GILL, C., "Galen and the Stoics: what each could learn from the other about embodied psychology", in D. FREDE and R. BURKHARD (eds.), *Body and soul in ancient philosophy*, pp. 409-423, Berlin.

GILL, C.; WHITMARSH, T. and WILKINS, J. (eds.), *Galen and the world of knowledge*. Cambridge.

GLEASON, M., "Shock and awe: the performance dimension of Galen's anatomical demonstrations", in C. GILL; T. WHITMARSH and J. WILKINS, (eds.), *Galen and the world of knowledge*, pp. 85-114, Cambridge.

GOUREVITCH , D., *La bibliographie scientifique de Galien: l'exemple de Soranos*. Rennes.

— "Il simulatore vorrebbe ingannare il medico: (secondo Galeno e altre fonti)", *QRO* 2, pp. 92-100.

HANKINSON, R.J., "Galen on the limits of knowledge", in C. GILL; T. WHITMARSH and J. WILKINS, (eds.), *Galen and the world of knowledge*, pp. 206-242, Cambridge.

— "Medicine and the science of soul", *Can Bull Med Hist*. 26.1, pp. 129-154.

IAVAZZO, C.R. et al., "The breast: from Ancient Greek myths to Hippocrates and Galen", *Reprod Biomed Online* 19.2, pp. 51-54.

JONES, C. P., "Books and libraries in a newly-discovered treatise of Galen", *JRA* 22.1, pp. 390-397.

JOUANNA, J., "Anonyme, «*Sur les quatre éléments*»: (Laur. plut. 75.19, fol. 26v-27r): publication d'un nouveau témoignage sur la chronobiologie quotidienne des quatre humeurs", *Galenos* 3, pp. 75-89.

KAPLAN, E.L. et al., "History of the recurrent laryngeal nerve: from Galen to Lahey", *World J Surg*. 33.3, pp. 386-393.

KARAMANOU, M.; ANDROUTSOS, G. and DIAMANTIS, A., "Cancer and Roman medicine", *J BUON*. 14.3, pp. 537-540.

KÖNIG, J., "Conventions of prefatory self-presentation in Galen's «*On the order of my own books*»", in C. GILL; T. WHITMARSH and J. WILKINS, (eds.), *Galen and the world of knowledge*, pp. 35-58, Cambridge.

LAMI, A., “Il nuovo Galeno e il fr. 964 di Euripide”, *Galenos* 3, pp. 11-19.

LEITH, D., “The qualitative status of the «onkoi» in Asclepiades’ theory of matter”, *OSAPh* 36, pp. 283-320.

LLOYD, G. E. R., “Galen’s un-Hippocratic case-histories”, in C. GILL; T. WHITMARSH and J. WILKINS, (eds.), *Galen and the world of knowledge*, pp. 115-131, Cambridge.

LÓPEZ FÉREZ. J.A., “Algunas notas de Galeno sobre la enseñanza y el aprendizaje de la medicina”, *Nova Tellus* 27.1, pp. 59-108.

LÓPEZ FIGUEROA, L., “La “*Epistola peri hereseon*” y el prólogo de comentario al tratado galénico “*De Sectis*””, *Galenos* 3, pp. 91-106.

MANETTI, D., “Galen and Hippocratic medicine: language and practice”, in C. GILL; T. WHITMARSH and J. WILKINS, (eds.), *Galen and the world of knowledge*, pp. 157-174, Cambridge.

— “Anonymus Londiniensis “*De Medicina*” (P. BR. LIBR. INV. 137) XVII 21-22. Collocazione di un frammento “*incertae sedis*””, *Galenos* 3, pp. 39-43.

NISSAN, E., “Deadly flowers and lethal plants: a theme in folklore, fiction and metaphoric imagery”, *Fabula* 50.3-4, pp. 293-311.

NISSEN, C., *Entre Asclépios et Hippocrate. Étude des cultes guérriseurs et des médecins en Carie*. Liege.

NUTTON, V., “Galen’s library”, in C. GILL; T. WHITMARSH and J. WILKINS, (eds.), *Galen and the world of knowledge*, pp. 19-34, Cambridge.

— “Biographical accounts of Galen, 1340-1660”, in T. RÜTTEN (ed.), *Geschichte der Medizingeschichtsschreibung: Historiographie unter dem Diktat literarischer Gattungen von der Antike bis zur Aufklärung*, pp. 201-232, Remscheid.

ROSE, F.C., “Cerebral localization in antiquity”, *J Hist Neurosci*. 18.3, pp. 239-247.

ROSELLI, A., “κάτθανε καὶ Πάτροκλος: un’interpretazione delle testimonianze su Callianatte Erofileo”, *Galenos* 3, pp. 69-74.

— “Due manoscritti medici greci nelle biblioteche di Sofia”, *Galenos* 3, pp. 177-180.

RÜTTEN, T., *Geschichte der Medizingeschichtsschreibung: Historiographie unter dem Diktat literarischer Gattungen von der Antike bis zur Aufklärung*. Remscheid.

SABBATANI, S. and FIORINO, S., “The Antonine Plague and the decline of the Roman Empire”, *Infez Med*. 17.4, pp. 261-275.

SANTANA HENRÍQUEZ, G., “La terminología médica sobre los dolores de cabeza en Galeno”, *Philologica canariensia* 14-15, pp. 279-296.

SCHÄFER, D., "«*Exemplum historiae naturalis*»: zur Funktion von Beispielen für ein hohes Alter in der diätetischen Literatur der Renaissance und der frühen Neuzeit", in T. RÜTTEN (ed.), *Geschichte der Medizingeschichtsschreibung: Historiographie unter dem Diktat literarischer Gattungen von der Antike bis zur Aufklärung*, pp. 265-293, Remscheid.

SHKLAR, G. and BRACKETT, C.A., "Galen on oral anatomy", *J Hist Dent*. 57.1, pp. 24-28.

STEGER, F., "Altern im Leben: Alterstopoi in der antiken Medizin ?", in D. ELM et al. (eds.), *Alterstopoi: das Wissen von den Lebensaltern in Literatur, Kunst und Theologie*, pp. 101-112, Berlin.

THADEUSZ, F., "Griff in die Wunde: der gelehrte Arzt Galen nutzte besondere Tricks Recueil: Das Ende des Römischen Reiches", in J. SALTZWEDEL (ed.), *Das Ende des Römischen Reiches: Verfall und Untergang einer Weltmacht*, pp. 192-196, Munich.

TIELEMAN, T., "Galen and the Stoics, or *The art of not naming*", in C. GILL; T. WHITMARSH and J. WILKINS, (eds.), *Galen and the world of knowledge*, pp. 282-299, Cambridge.

TUCCI, P.L., "Antium, the Palatium and the Domus Tiberiana again", *JRA* 22.1, pp. 398-401.

VASILIADIS, E.S.; GRIVAS, T.B. and KASPIRIS, A., "Historical overview of spinal deformities in ancient Greece", *Scoliosis* 25, pp. 4-6.

VELA TEJADA, J., ""Koiné" y aticismo en Galeno, "*De antidotis*": datos para un estudio lingüístico", *CFC(G)* 19, pp. 41-61.

VON STADEN, H., "Staging the past, staging oneself: Galen on Hellenistic exegetical traditions", in C. GILL; T. WHITMARSH and J. WILKINS, (eds.), *Galen and the world of knowledge*, pp. 132-156, Cambridge.

YEO, I.S., "Heat and Fever in ancient Greek physiology", *Uisahak* 18.2, pp. 189-203.

ZAGO, G., "Per l'emendazione di tre luoghi galenico-posidoniani", *SIFC* 7.2, pp. 241-247.

ZIPSER, B., "Deleted text in a manuscript: Galen «*On the eye*» and the Marc. Gr. 276", *Galenos* 3, pp. 107-112.

2008

ALEXANDER, L., "The passions in Galen and the novels of Chariton and Xenophon", in J.T. FITZGERALD (ed.), *Passions and moral progress in Greco-Roman thought*, pp. 175-197, London.

ANDÒ, V., "Female erotic dreams and female seed in ancient Greek medicine", *MedSec* 21.2, pp. 663-691.

ARATA, L., "Due emmenagoghi in Sulle malattie femminili I 74", *Galenos* 2, pp. 11-14.

AZIZI, M.H.; NAYERNOURI, T. and AZIZI, F., "A brief history of the discovery of the circulation of blood in the human body", *Arch Iran Med.* 11.3, pp. 345-350.

BARTOLI, V., "L'idropisia di maestro Adamo en Inferno XXX. Importanza della dottrina umorale di Galeno nel medioevo", *Tenzone* 8, pp. 11-29.

BOUDON-MILLOT, V., "Galien de Pergame témoin de son temps: l'acculturation de la médicine grecque à la société romaine du IIe siècle de n.è.", *Semitica & Classica* 1, pp. 71-80

— "Un étudiant sans école, un maître sans disciples: l'example paradoxal de Galien de Pergame", in H.HUGONNARD-ROCHE (ed.), *L'enseignement supérieur dans les mondes antiques et médiévaux. Aspects institutionnels, juridiques et pédagogiques*, pp. 265-282, Paris.

CHRISTOPOULOU-ALETRA, H. and PAPAVRAMIDOU, N., "'Diabetes as described by Byzantine writers from the fourth to the ninth century AD: the Graeco-Roman influence", *Diabetologia* 51.5, pp. 892-896.

COSTANZA, S., "Galeno, «*De dignotione ex insomniis*»: nuove fonti della tradizione manoscritta medievale", *RPL* 11, pp. 136-142.

CULLYER, H.C., "Chrysippus on Achilles: the evidence of Galen *De placitis Hippocratis et Platonis* 4.6-7", *CQ* 58.2, pp. 537-546.

DEBRU, A., "Physiology", in R.J. HANKINSON (ed.), *The Cambridge Companion to Galen*, pp. 263-282, Cambridge.

— "Les enseignements de la torpille dans la médecine antique", in I. BOEHM and P. LUCCIONI (ed.), *Le médecin initié par l'animal: animaux et médecine dans l'Antiquité grecque et latine*, pp. 39-48, Lyon.

DRIZIS, T.J., "Medical ethics in a writing of Galen", *Acta Med Hist Adriat.* 6.2, pp. 333-336.

EIJK, P. J., "Therapeutics", in R.J. HANKINSON (ed.), *The Cambridge Companion to Galen*, pp. 283-303, Cambridge.

FISCHER, K.-D. et al., "Congetture inedite sui testi medici", *Galenos* 2, pp. 135-142.

FITZGERALD, J.T. (ed.), *Passions and moral progress in Greco-Roman thought*. London.

FLEMMING, R., "Commentary", in R.J. HANKINSON (ed.), *The Cambridge Companion to Galen*, pp. 323-354, Cambridge.

FORTUNA, S., "Pietro d'Abano e le traduzioni latine di Galeno", *MedSec* 20.2, pp. 447-463.

— "Girolamo Mercuriale editore di Galeno", in A. ARCANGELI and V. NUTTON (eds.), *Girolamo Mercuriale. Medicina e cultura nell'europa del cinquecento*, pp. 217-231, Florence.

— "L'interruzione della gravidanza nel mondo antico", *Lettere dalla Facoltà, Bollettino della Facoltà di Medicina e Chirurgia dell'Università Politecnica delle Marche* 11, p. 43.

— "Galeno e il «*Timeo*» di Platone (91a)", in V.V.A.A., *Filologia, papirologia, storia dei testi: giornate di studio in onore di Antonio Carlini*, pp. 273-288, Pisa.

FRAMPTON, M., *Voluntary animal motion from Greek antiquity to the Latin Middle Ages, 400 B.C.-A.D. 1300*. Chicago.

GAROFALO, I., "Gli scoli al «*De sectis*» e all' «*Ad Glauconem*» nel Parisinus suppl. gr. 634", *Galenos* 2, pp. 61-105.

— "Povertà nel galenismo e in Galeno", *Mediterraneo Antico* 10.1-2, pp. 269-277.

GILL, C., "Die antike medizinische Tradition: die körperliche Basis emotionaler Dispositionen", in H. LANDWEER and U. RENZ (eds.), *Klassische Emotionstheorien: von Platon bis Wittgenstein*, pp. 97-120, Berlin.

GONZÁLEZ-GONZÁLEZ, J.J.; SANZ-ALVAREZ, L. and GARCÍA BERNARDO, C., "Obesity in the history of surgery", *Cir Esp*. 84.4, pp. 188-195.

GRIMAUDO, S., *Difendere la salute: igiene e disciplina del soggetto nel «De sanitate tuenda» di Galeno*. Naples.

— "Galeno, «*L'ordine dei suoi libri*» e i destinatari del trattato di «Igiene»: (*De ord. libr. suor.* II 13)", *Galenos* 2, pp. 57-60.

HAAS, C., "Silphium from Cyrenaica, an extinct medicinal plant", *Bull Acad Natl Med*. 192.1, pp. 153-160.

HANKINSON, R.J. (ed.), *The Cambridge Companion to Galen*. Cambridge.

— "The man and his work", in R.J. HANKINSON (ed.), *The Cambridge Companion to Galen*, pp. 1-33, Cambridge.

— "Psychology", in R.J. HANKINSON (ed.), *The Cambridge Companion to Galen*, pp. 184-209, Cambridge.

— "Philosophy of Nature", in R.J. HANKINSON (ed.), *The Cambridge Companion to Galen*, pp. 210-241, Cambridge.

— "Epistemology", in R.J. HANKINSON (ed.), *The Cambridge Companion to Galen*, pp. 157-183, Cambridge.

HEARY, R.F. and MADHAVAN, K., "The history of spinal deformity", *Neurosurgery* 63.3, pp. 5-15.

HERNÁNDEZ GONZÁLEZ, J.P., "El Doctor López Canario y sus comentarios al *De temperamentis* de Galeno (1565)", *Estudios Canarios* 50-51, pp. 677-688.

KOVACIC, F., "Intensität der Elementarqualitäten nach Galen", *Traditio* 63, pp. 1-44.

LEGUTKO, J. et al., "The history of treatment of groin hernia", *Folia Med Cracov.* 49.1-2, pp. 57-74.

LEITH, D., "The «*diatritus*» and therapy in Graeco-Roman medicine", *CQ* 58.2, pp. 581-600.

LLOYD, G. E. R., "Galen and his contemporaries", in R.J. HANKINSON (ed.), *The Cambridge Companion to Galen*, pp. 34-48, Cambridge.

MANETTI, D., "*Londiniensis medicus*", in P. KEYSER and G.L. IRBY-MASSIE (eds.), *The Encyclopedia of Ancient natural Scientists*, pp. 517-518, London.

MARTÍNEZ, F. and DECUADRO SÁENZ. G., "Claudio Galeno y los ventrículos cerebrales: Parte I, los antecedentes", *Neurocirugía* 19.1, pp. 58-65.

MATTERN, S. P., *Galen and the rhetoric of healing*. Baltimore.

— "Galen's Ideal Patient", in L. CILLIERS (ed.), *Asklepios. Studies on Ancient Medicine,* pp. 116-130, Bloemfontein.

MESTRE, F., "Uso y abuso de los libros en un mundo libresco: algunos ejemplos griegos de la época imperial", *Faventia* 30.1-2, pp. 297-313.

MORISON, B., "Logic", in R.J. HANKINSON (ed.), *The Cambridge Companion to Galen*, pp. 66-115, Cambridge.

— "Language", in R.J. HANKINSON (ed.), *The Cambridge Companion to Galen*, pp. 116-156, Cambridge.

MÜLKE, M., "«*Primus scriptor*»: ein übersehener Akteur antiker Buch- und Überlieferungsgeschichte?", in S. HEILEN (ed.), *In pursuit of «Wissenschaft»: Festschrift für William M. Calder III zum 75. Geburtstag*, pp. 315-325, Hildesheim-New York.

MÜLLER, R., *Gelassenheit: Analysen zu Galen und Seneca im Horizont pädagogischer Anthropologie*. Münster.

NUTTON, V., "The fortunes of Galen", in R.J. HANKINSON (ed.), *The Cambridge Companion to Galen*, pp. 355-390, Cambridge.

— "The manuscripts of the Latin Galen and a Quotation from *De Humoribus*", in V. BOUDOT; A. GUARDASOLE and C. MAGDELAINE (eds.), *La science médicale antique. Nouveaux regards*, pp. 339-352, Paris.

— "Ancient Mediterranean pharmacology and cultural transfer", *European Review* 16, pp. 211-217.

— "Greek medical astrology and the boundaries of medicine", in A. AKASOY; C. BURNETT and R. YOELI-TLALIM, *Astro-Medicine. Astrology and Medicine, East and West*, pp. 17-31, Florence.

PALMIERI, N. (ed.), *L'ars medica (tegni) de Galien: lectures antiques et médiévales*. Saint-Étienne.

PERILLI, L., "Su Esichio e i cosiddetti «*frammenti*» del «*Glossario ippocratico*» di Erotiano", *Galenos* 2, pp. 35-55.

PINO CAMPOS, L.M. and HERNÁNDEZ GONZÁLEZ, J.P., "En torno al significado original del vocablo griego «*epidemía*» y su identificación con el latino «*pestis*»", *Dynamis* 28, pp. 199-215.

PORMANN, P.E., "Case notes and clinicians. Galen's commentary on the hippocratic epidemics in the arabic tradition", *Arab Sci Philos* 18.2, pp. 247-284.

ROCCA, J., "Anatomy", in R.J. HANKINSON (ed.), *The Cambridge Companion to Galen*, pp. 242-262, Cambridge.

SABRINA, G., *Difendere la salute: igiene e disciplina del soggetto nel de sanitate tuenda di Galeno*. Naples.

SOMMEREY, K.M., "Die Chora von Pergamon: Studien zu Grenzen, Siedlungsstruktur und Wirtschaft", *MDAI(I)* 58, pp. 135-170.

TIELEMAN, T., "Methodology", in R.J. HANKINSON (ed.), *The Cambridge Companion to Galen*, pp. 49-65, Cambridge.

TUCCI, P.L., "Galen's storeroom, Rome's libraries, and the fire of A.D. 192", *JRA* 21.1, pp. 133-149.

VOGT, S., "Drugs and pharmacology", in R.J. HANKINSON (ed.), *The Cambridge Companion to Galen*, pp. 304-322, Cambridge.

WALLER, J., "Lessons from the history of medicine", *J Invest Surg*. 21.2, pp. 53-56.

WILKINS, J., "Animals in the Romano-Greek culture of the second century A.D.", in A. ALEXANDRIDIS; M. WILD and L. WINKLER-HORACEK (eds.), *Mensch und Tier in der Antike: Grenzziehung und Grenzüberschreitung*, pp. 315-328, Wiesbaden.

2007

ANNESE, P., "L'indice del «*De naturalibus facultatibus*» nel Laurentianus 74.5", *Galenos* 1, pp. 219-220.

ARONSON, S.M., "Galen and the causes of disease", *Med Health R I.* 90.12, p. 375.

BERRYMAN, S.A., "Teleology without tears: Aristotle and the role of mechanistic conceptions of organisms", *CJPh* 37.3, pp. 351-370.

BOYLAN, M., "Galen: on blood, the pulse and the arteries", *JHB* 40.2, pp. 207-230.

BRAVO GARCÍA, A., "En torno al control que el alma no ejerce sobre el cuerpo en ciertas ocasiones: (a propósito de Platón, Plutarco y Agustín, con una ojeada a la medicina griega)", in A. BERNABÉ and I. RODRÍGUEZ ALFAGEME (eds.), *Φίλου σκιά: studia philologiae in honorem Rosae Aguilar ab amicis et sodalibus dicata*, pp. 109-125, Madrid.

BROWN, R.T., "Galen: developer of the reversal design?", *Behav Anal.* 30.1, pp. 31-35.

CEREZO MAGÁN, M., "El símil como expediente paradigmático en "*Sobre la utilidad de las partes del cuerpo humano*" de Galeno", *EC* 49, pp. 27-46.

CRUZ-COKE, M.R., "A journey to the foundations of classical medicine", *Rev Med Chil.* 135.8, pp. 1076-1081.

DEBRU, A., *Galen on pharmacology, philosophy, history and medicine*. Leiden.

DONINI, P., "Seneca e Galeno sulla struttura proposizionale delle passioni in Crisippo", *RSF* 62.3, pp. 431-452.

ESCARPA, D., "La salud y la enfermedad en el templo de Asclepio", in J.L. GONZÁLEZ RECIO (ed.), *Átomos, almas y estrellas: estudios sobre la ciencia griega*, pp. 201-236, Madrid.

FLEMMING, R., "Galen's imperial order of knowledge", in J. KÖNIG and T. WHITMARSH (eds.), *Ordering knowledge in the Roman Empire*, pp. 241-277, Cambridge.

GARCÍA NOVO, E., "Pietro d'Ábano y su traducción del tratado de Galeno «*De inaequali intemperie*»", in A. BERNABÉ and I. RODRÍGUEZ ALFAGEME (eds.), *Φίλου σκιά: studia philologiae in honorem Rosae Aguilar ab amicis et sodalibus dicata*, pp. 223-234, Madrid.

GARCÍA VALVERDE, J.M., "El galenismo crítico de Girolamo Cardano: análisis de la presencia de Galeno en el "*De inmortalitate Animorum*"", Asclepio 1, pp. 35-64.

GAROFALO, I., "La traduzione araba del «*De sectis*» e il sommario degli Alessandrini", *Galenos* 1, pp. 191-210.

GAROFALO, I. et al., "Congetture inedite sui testi medici", *Galenos* 1, pp. 221-228.

GILL, C., "Galen and the Stoics: mortal enemies or blood brothers?", *Phronesis* 52.1, pp. 88-120.

GRUNERT, P.; CHARALAMPAKI, P. and AYYAD, A., "Concept and treatment of hydrocephalus in the Greco-Roman and early Arabic medicine", *Minim Invasive Neurosurg*. 50.5, pp. 253-264.

IERACI BIO, A.M., "«Dihaireseis» relative all'«*Ars Medica*» di Galeno nel Neap. Orat. gr. CF 2.11 (olim XXII-1)", *Galenos* 1, pp. 149-161.

JU, A.E., "Chrysippus on nature and soul in animals", *CQ* 57.1, pp. 97-108.

KEEMAN, J.N., "Bloodletting; a popular form of treatment that disappeared", *Ned Tijdschr Geneeskd*. 151.3, pp. 206-211.

KEMP, W., "The earliest known French translation of Galen (ca. 1530) at the Osler library", *Osler Libr Newsl*. 107, pp. 1-5.

KÖNIG, J. and WHITMARSH, T. (eds.), *Ordering knowledge in the Roman Empire*. Cambridge.

KSHETTRY, V.R.; MINDEA, S.A. and BATJER, H.H., "The management of cranial injuries in antiquity and beyond", *Neurosurg Focus*. 23.1, p. 8.

LEHOUX, D., "Observers, objects, and the embedded eye or Seeing and Knowing in Ptolemy and Galen", *Isis* 98.3, pp. 447-467.

LO PRESTI, R., "*La medicina alla prova. Verso una pragmatica della ricerca biomedica*", in V. ANDÒ and G. NICOLACI (eds.), *Processo alla prova. Modelli e pratiche di verifica dei saperi*, pp. 235-263, Rome.

LÓPEZ SACO, J. O., "Una aproximación a la «demencia» en la Roma y el Oriente Antiguo", *Praesentia* 8 (http://vereda.saber.ula.ve/sol/praesentia8/julio.htm).

LÓPEZ SALVÁ, M., "Galeno: del cuerpo, el alma, el espíritu y el sistema conectivo", in A. BERNABÉ and I. RODRÍGUEZ ALFAGEME (eds.), *Φίλου σκιά: studia philologiae in honorem Rosae Aguilar ab amicis et sodalibus dicata*, pp. 205-221, Madrid.

MISSIOS, S., "Hippocrates, Galen, and the uses of trepanation in the ancient classical world", *Neurosurg Focus* 23.1, p. 11.

NUTTON, V., "«*De motibus liquidis*» and the medieval Latin Galen", *Galenos* 1, pp. 163-173.

— "Greco-Roman medicine and the Greek Papyri", in H. FROSCHAUER and C. RÖÖMER (eds.), *Zwischen Magie und Wissenschaft. Ärzte und Heilkunst in den Papyri aus Ägypten,* pp. 5-12, Wien.

— "Galen in Byzantium", in M. GRÜNBART et al. (eds.), *Material Culture and Well-being in Byzantium*, pp. 171-176, Wien.

PAPAVRAMIDOU, N. and CHRISTOPOULOU-ALETRA, H., "Diabetes and the "Natural Faculties" in the Galenic treatises", *Hormones* 6.2, pp. 157-159.

PETIT, C., "Gadaldini's library", *Mnemosyne* 60.1, pp. 132-138.

RAIOLA, T., "Una nota sul «*De propriis placitis*» di Galeno", *AION(filol)* 29, pp. 137-139.

ROCCA, J., "W.L.H. Duckworth (1870-1956) and his translation of Galen's *Anatomical Procedures*", *J Med Biogr.* 15.3, pp. 134-138.

ROSELLI, A., "Memoria e sommatoria nel processo cognitivo: con edizione di Galeno, *comm. in Hipp. off. med.* XVIII B 650,8-652,13 Kühn", *Galenos* 1, pp. 73-85.

SAKAI, T., "Historical evolution of anatomical terminology from ancient to modern", *Anat Sci Int.* 82.2, pp. 65-81.

SCHIEFSKY, M., "Galen's teleology and functional explanation", *OSAPh* 33, pp. 369-400.

STROHMAIER, G., "La longévité de Galien et les deux places de son tombeau", in V. BOUDON-MILLOT; A. GUARDASOLE and C. MAGDELAINE (eds.), *La science médicale antique. Nouveaux regards, Études réunies en l'honneur de J. Jouanna*, pp. 393-403, Paris.

TODMAN, D., "Galen (129-199)", *J Neurol.* 254.7, pp. 975-976.

TOMEY, M.I.; KOMOTAR, R.J. and MOCCO, J., "Herophilus, Erasistratus, Aretaeus, and Galen: ancient roots of the Bell-Magendie Law", *Neurosurg Focus.* 23.1, p. 12.

TUOMINEN, M., "Heaps, experience, and method: on the sorites argument in ancient medicine", *HPhQ* 24.2, pp. 109-125.

VIALE, G.L., "The surgical approach to the posterior cranial fossa according to Galen", *Neurosurgery.* 61.2, pp. 399-403.

WILKINS, J. B., "Galen and Athenaeus in the Hellenistic library", in J. KÖNIG and T. WHITMARSH (eds.), *Ordering knowledge in the Roman Empire*, pp. 69-87, Cambridge.

2006

ANDRÉ, J.-M., *La médecine à Rome*. Paris.

BALIN, P., "Le médecin à l'écoute des rêves", *Incontri triestini di filologia classica* 4, pp. 49-58.

— "Apprendre à regarder", in J. BOULOGNE and A. DRIZENKO (eds.), *L'enseignement de la médecine selon Galien*, Lille, pp. 79-86.

BARTELS, E.M.; SWADDLING, J. and HARRISON, A.P., "An ancient Greek pain remedy for athletes", *Pain Pract.* 6.3, pp. 212-218.

BOUDON-MILLOT, V., "Figures du maître chez Galien", in J. BOULOGNE and A. DRIZENKO (eds.), *L'enseignement de la médecine selon Galien*, pp. 15-30, Lille.

BOULOGNE, J., "La thérapie des plaies selon Galien. Un enseignement à base de polémique (*De methodo medendi, III-VI*)", in J. BOULOGNE and A. DRIZENKO (eds.), *L'enseignement de la médecine selon Galien*, pp. 121-142, Lille.

BOULOGNE, J and DRIZENKO, A. (eds.), *L'enseignement de la médecine selon Galien*. Lille.

BRABANT, D., "Persönliche Gotteserfahrung und religiöse Gruppe: die Therapeutai des Asklepios in Pergamon", in A. GUTSFELD and K. DIETRICH-ALEX (eds.), *Vereine, Synagogen und Gemeinden im kaiserzeitlichen Kleinasien*, pp. 61-75, Tübingen.

CORVISIER, J. N., "Les commentaires hippocratiques comme moyen d'enseignement de la médicice", in J. BOULOGNE and A. DRIZENKO (eds.), *L'enseignement de la médecine selon Galien*, pp. 111-120, Lille.

DEAN-JONES, L.A., "Galen on the brain: review article", *Apeiron* 39.3, pp. 289-292.

DRIZENKO, A., "Dissection et vivisection dans l'enseignement physiologique de Galien, l'exemple du *rete mirabile*", in J. BOULOGNE and A. DRIZENKO (eds.), *L'enseignement de la médecine selon Galien*, pp. 67-78, Lille.

ENDRESS, G., "Kopf und Herz, Geist und Seele in den Wissenschaftsparadigmen des arabisch-islamischen Mittelalters", in K. PHILIPOWSKI and A. PRIOR (eds.), *«Anima» und «Sêl»: Darstellungen und Systematisierungen von Seele im Mittelalter*, pp. 3-20, Berlin.

FORTUNA, S., "Sui manoscritti greci di Galeno appartenuti a Nicolò Leoniceno e al cardinale Bessarione", in G. FIACCADORI; A. GATTI and S. MAROTTA (eds.), *«In partibus Clius»: scritti in onore di Giovanni Pugliese Carratelli*, pp. 189-211, Naples.

FORTUNA, S. and RAIA, A., "*Corrigenda* and *addenda* to Diels' *Galenica* by Richard J. Durling. III. Manuscripts and editions", *Traditio* 61, pp. 1-30.

GAROFALO, I., "L' enseignement de l'anatomie chez Galien", in J. BOULOGNE and A. DRIZENKO (eds.), *L'enseignement de la médecine selon Galien*, pp. 59-66, Lille.

GOUVERITCH, D., "Pourquoi des récits de cas? *Ad introducendos*", in J. BOULOGNE and A. DRIZENKO (eds.), *L'enseignement de la médecine selon Galien*, pp. 87-110, Lille.

HAAS, C., "The Antonine plague", *Bull Acad Natl Med.* 190.4-5, pp. 1093-1098.

JOUANNA, J., "Ne pas s'étonner chez Hippocrate et chez Galien", in J. BOULOGNE and A. DRIZENKO (eds.), *L'enseignement de la médecine selon Galien*, Lille, pp. 143-156.

KANZ, F. and GROSSCHMIDT, K., "Head injuries of Roman Gladiators", *Forensic Science International* 160.2-3, pp. 207-216.

LAES, C., "Galen on the division of childhood: some reconsiderations", *RSA* 36, pp. 229-240.

LEJAVITZER, A., "Algunas recetas médicas en el «*De re coquinaria*» de Apicio", *Nova Tellus* 24 (1), pp. 123-139.

LEVET, J.-P., "Logique et pédagogie médicale chez Galien", in J. BOULOGNE and A. DRIZENKO (eds.), *L'enseignement de la médecine selon Galien*, Lille, pp. 31-42.

LÓPEZ PÉREZ, M., "La transmisión a la Edad Media de la ciencia médica clásica", *A&Cr* 23, pp. 899-911.

LÓPEZ PIÑERO, J.Mª., "Galeno de Pérgamo (ca. 130-200)", *Mente y cerebro* 22, pp. 8-11.

LUJÁN MARTÍNEZ, E.A., "Cuatro notas críticas", in E. CALDERÓN DORDA; M.A. MORALES ORTIZ and M. VALVERDE SÁNCHEZ (eds.), *«Koinòs lógos»: homenaje al profesor José García López*, pp. 543-549, Murcia.

MACLEAN, I., "The "sceptical crisis" reconsidered: Galen, rational medicine and the *libertas philosophandi*", *Early Sci Med.* 11.3, pp. 247-274.

MANETTI, D., "La terminologie du livre: à propos des emplois d'*huphos* et *edaphos* dans deux passages de Galien", *REG* 119, pp. 157-171.

MARGANNE, M.-H., "Étiquettes des médicaments, listes de drogues, prescriptions et réceptaires dans l' Égypte gréco-romaine et byzantine", in F.COLLARD and E. SAMANA (eds.), *Pharmacopoles et apothicaires. Les pharmaciens de l'Antiquité au Grand Siècle*, pp. 59-73, Paris.

McVAUGH, M.R., "Niccolo da Reggio's translations of Galen and their reception in France", *Early Sci Med.* 11.3, pp. 275-301.

MOOG, F. and SCHÄFER, D., "Die Demenzkasuistiken in der «*Gerontologia*» (1705) des Theodosius Schöpffer: ein Vergleich mit überlieferten Darstellungen aus Literatur und Medizin", *NLJ* 8, pp. 201-226.

MUGGITTU, V., "Sul significato del termine ἄορτρον in [Ippocrate], Malattie II, 54a", *FAM* 30-31, pp. 21-32.

NIETO IBÁÑEZ, J.Mª., "Galeno: sinopsis de su propia obra sobre pulsos", *Minerva* 19, pp. 336-338.

PINO CAMPOS, L.M., "Observaciones al tratado de Galeno *Acerca de la diferencia de los pulsos*", *Fortunatae* 17, pp. 99-116.

RECEK, C., "Historical review of opinions on the nature of varicose veins and leg ulcers and their treatment", *Rozhl Chir.* 85.12, pp. 641-645.

ROCCA, J., "«Plato will tell you»: Galen's use of the «*Phaedrus*» in *De Placitis Hippocratis et Platonis* IX", in H.A.S. TARRANT and D.C. BALTZLY (eds.), *Reading Plato in Antiquity*, pp. 49-59, London.

SKODA, F., "L' enseignement par Galien des noms et des choses: lexicographie et modernité", in J. BOULOGNE and A. DRIZENKO (eds.), *L'enseignement de la médecine selon Galien*, pp. 43-58, Lille.

SWAIN, S., "Beyond the limits of Greek biography: Galen from Alexandria to the Arabs", in B.C. MCGING and J.M. MOSSMAN (eds.), *The limits of Ancient Biography*, pp. 395-433, London and Swansea.

TOUWAIDE, A., "The kidney from Galen to Vesalius -a first approach", *J Nephrol.* 19, pp. 4-8.

WILSON, M.C. and DEMETRA, G., "Anonymi, «*De Decubitu*»: contexts of rationality", *Mouseion* 6.3, pp. 439-452.

ZUÑIGA, J.M., "There's something about Galen", *IAPAC* 12.9, pp. 292-293.

2005

BACALEXI, D., "Female responsibilities: midwives, nurses and mothers in the works of some antique and Renaissance physicians", *Gesnerus* 62.1-2, pp. 5-32.

BARNES, J., "What is a disjunction?", in D. FREDE and B. INWOOD (eds.), *Language and learning: philosophy of language in the Hellenistic Age*, pp. 274-298, Cambridge.

BARRAS, V., "Le «Galen's touch»: peau, objet et sujet dans le système médical galénien", *Micrologus* 13, pp. 55-73.

BIEGANOWSKI, L., "Galen from Pergamon (130-200) –views on ophthalmology. Part II –anatomic description of the eye", *Klin Oczna.* 107.1-3, pp. 173-176.

BONED COLERA, P., "El texto dentro del texto: Filón, un poeta alejandrino en Galeno", in A. ALVAR EZQUERRA et al. (eds.), *Actas del XI Congreso Español de Estudios Clásicos*, pp. 253-260, Madrid.

BOUDON-MILLOT, V., "A great and forgotten physician: Galen of Pergamon", *Rev Prat.* 55.16, pp. 1850-1853.

CANTOR, D., "Between Galen, Geddes, and the Gael: Arthur Brock, modernity, and medical humanism in early-twentieth-century Scotland", *J Hist Med Allied Sci*. 60.1, pp. 1-41.

CLARK, G., "The health of the spiritual athlete", in H. KING (ed.), *Health in Antiquity*, pp. 216-229, London.

DIAMANDOPOULOS, A. and GOUDAS, P., "You can't make a monkey out of us: Galen and genetics versus Darwin", *Vesalius* 11.2, pp. 61-63.

EIJK, P.J., *Medicine and Philosophy in Classical Antiquity. Doctors and Philosophers on Nature, Soul, Health and Disease*. Cambridge.

ELLIOT, C.J., *Galen, Rome and the Second Sophistic*. Unpublished PhD.

FORTUNA, S., "Alle origini della medicina moderna", in G.C. BOJANI; M. PATTI and M. TAGLIABRACCI (eds.), *L'arte della cura. Antichi libri di medicina, botanica e vasi da farmacia*, pp. 17-20, Urbania.

— "Galeno Latino, 1490-1533", *MedSec* 17.2, pp. 469-505.

— "La malattia nel mondo antico: da Ippocrate a Galeno", in V.V.A.A., *Temi di medicina antica*, pp. 15-26, L'Aquila.

GADEBUSH BONDIO, M., *Medizinische Ästhetik: Kosmetik und plastische Chirurgie zwischen Antike und früher Neuzeit*. Munich.

GAROFALO, I., "Aspetti della tradizione dei testi medici antichi", V.V.A.A. *Temi di medicina antica*, pp. 55-61, L'Aquila.

— "Galen's Commentary on Hippocrates' *De Humoribus*", in P.J. EIJK (ed.), *Hippocrates in context*, pp. 445-456 Leiden.

GILL, C., "Tragic fragments, ancient philosophers and the fragmented self", in F. MCHARDY; J. ROBSON and D. HARVEY (eds.), *Lost dramas of classical Athens: Greek tragic fragments*, pp. 151-172, Exeter.

HIERONYMUS, F., *Theophrast und Galen - Celsus und Paracelsus: Medizin, Naturphilosophie und Kirchenreform im Basler Buchdruck bis zum Dreissigjährigen Krieg*. Basilea.

KLEIN-FRANKE, F. and MING, Z., "How Galen's "sixteen books" came to China in the tenth century AD", *Am J Chin Med*. 33 (2), pp. 339-342.

LLOYD, G.E.R., "Mathematics as a Model in Galen", in R.W. SHARPLES (ed.), *Philosophy and Sciences in Antiquity*, pp. 110-130, Aldershot.

LORUSSO, V., "Nuovi frammenti di Galeno (*In Hp. Epid. VI Comm.* VII ; *In Plat. Tim. Comm.*)", *ZPE* 152, pp. 43-56.

MANETTI, D., "Galeno e la definizione del lessico medico", in V.V.A.A., *Temi di medicina antica*, pp. 63-71, L'Aquila.

MOOG, F.P.; KARENBERG, A. and MOLL, F., "The catheter and its use from Hippocrates to Galen", *J Urol.* 174.4, pp. 1196-1198.

NORN, S.; KRUSE, P.R. and KRUSE, E., "History of opium poppy and morphine", *Dan Medicinhist Arbog.* 33, pp. 171-184.

NUTTON, V., "The fatal embrace: Galen and the history of ancient medicine", *Sci Context.* 18.1, pp. 111-121.

OVERWIEN, O, "Einige Beobachtungen zur Überlieferung der Hippokratesschriften in der arabischen und griechischen Tradition", *Sudhoffs Archiv* 89.2, pp. 196-210.

PERILLI, L., "Cronaca di un'avventura editoriale: il «*Galeno*» di Aldo Manuzio e l'ombra di Erasmo", *GCFI* 1.3, pp. 422-432.

PINO CAMPOS, L.M., "Panorama general del conocimiento del pulso cardiovascular en Plutarco", in M. JUFRESA et al. (eds.), *Plutarc a la seva època: paideia i societat: actas del VIII simposio español sobre Plutarco*, pp. 109-115, Barcelona.

SANTANA HENRÍQUEZ, G., "El cuerpo en la medicina griega imperial: sobre los dolores de cabeza en Galeno", in E. PADORNO and G. SANTANA HENRÍQUEZ (eds.), *El cuerpo*, pp. 9-44, Las Palmas de Gran Canaria.

SCHOLTEN, C., "Welche Seele hat der Embryo?: Johannes Philoponos und die antike Embryologie", *VChr* 59.4, pp. 377-411.

STEFANI, C., "Alcune congetture al «*De propriorum animi cuiuslibet affectuum et peccatorum dignotione et curatione*» di Galeno", *SIFC* 3.2, pp. 251-255.

WILKINS, J. M., "Hygieia at dinner and at the symposium", in H. KING (ed.), *Health in Antiquity*, pp. 136 149, London.

YEO, I.S., "Hippocrates in the context of Galen: Galen's commentary on the classification of fevers in *Epidemics* VI", in P.J. EIJK (ed.), *Hippocrates in context*, pp. 433-443, Leiden.

2004

AGUILAR, R.Mª., "A Medea le duele la cabeza: comentario a Apolonio Rodio III", *CFC(G)* 14, pp. 761-765.

ALBY, J.C., "La concepción antropológica de la medicina hipocrática", *Enfoques* 16.1, pp. 5-29.

ALLEN, J., "Experience as a source and ground of theory in Epicureanism", *Apeiron* 37.4, pp. 89-106.

BACALEXI, D., "Trois traducteurs de Galien au XVIe siècle: Niccolò Leoniceno, Guillaume Cop, Leonhart Fuchs", in V. BOUDON-MILLOT and G. COBOLET (eds.), *Lire les médecins grecs à la Renaissance*, pp. 247-269, Paris.

BECKER, L. C., "Stoic emotion", in S.K. STRANGE and J. ZUPKO (eds.), *Stoicism: traditions and transformations*, pp. 250-275, Cambridge.

BIEGANOWSKI, L., "Galen of Pergamum (130-200), his views on ophthalmology (part I)", *Klin Oczna*. 106.4-5, pp. 706-710.

BOEHM, I., "Connaissance et diffusion du traité de Galien «*Des facultés naturelles*» à la Renaissance", in V. BOUDON-MILLOT and G. COBOLET (eds.), *Lire les médecins grecs à la Renaissance*, pp. 233-245, Paris.

CAVARRA, B., "Su alcune annotazioni di carattere medico contenute in un manoscritto greco (Ambr. C 222 inf., f. 40r)", *Aevum* 78.2, pp. 517-530.

CITRONI MARCHETTI, S., "I precetti paterni e le lezioni dei filosofi: Demea, il padre di Orazio ed altri padri e figli", *MD* 53, pp. 9-63.

DRIZENKO, A. "Jacques Dubois, dit Sylvius, traducteur et commentateur de Galien", in V. BOUDON-MILLOT and G. COBOLET (eds.), *Lire les médecins grecs à la Renaissance*, pp. 199-208, Paris.

FORTUNA, S., "Conoscere e riconoscere le malattie: da Ippocrate a Galeno", *L'Arco di Giano* 40, p. 9-18,

— "Libri e fondi antichi di medicina nelle biblioteche delle marche", in M. MEI (ed.), *Collectio Thesauri. Dalle marche tesori nascosti di un collezionismo illustre*, pp. 43-50, Florence.

— "La malattia nel mondo antico", *Bollettino della facoltà di medicina e chirurgia dell'università Politecnica delle Marche* 7, pp. 12-16.

GARCÍA NOVO, E., "Les éditions du traité de Galien «*De inaequali intemperie*» à la Renaissance", in V. BOUDON-MILLOT and G. COBOLET (eds.), *Lire les médecins grecs à la Renaissance*, pp. 187-198, Paris.

GAROFALO, I., "Agostino Gadaldini (1515-1575) et le Galien latin", in V. BOUDON-MILLOT and G. COBOLET (eds.), *Lire les médecins grecs à la Renaissance*, pp. 283-316, Paris.

GIL FERNÁNDEZ, L., "La diagnosis onírica de Galeno", *CFC(G)* 14, pp. 139-153.

GONZÁLEZ ECHEVARRÍA, F.M. and ANCÍN CHANDÍA, T., "La edición Lyonesa de la *Opera Omnia de Galeno* del impresor Jean Frellon (1548-1551) comentada por Miguel Serveto", in J. MARTÍNEZ PÉREZ (ed.), *La medicina ante el nuevo milenio: una perspectiva histórica*, pp. 645-657, Cuenca.

GOUDARD, P. and BARRAULT, D. (eds.), *Médecine du cirque: vingt siècles après Galien*. Vic-la-Gardiole.

GOUREVITCH, D., "L'insegnamento medico di Galeno: perché narra casi clinici?", *MedSec* 16.2, pp. 253-275.

GRAPPONE, A.G., "Galen's logic for medical diagnosis: a development", *Metalogicon* 17.1, pp. 25-32.

HUBY, P. M., "Elementary logic in the ancient world", *BICS* 47, pp. 119-128.

KARPOZILOS, A. and PAVLIDIS, N., "The treatment of cancer in Greek Antiquity", *Eur J Cancer* 40.14, pp. 2033-2040.

KUPREEVA, I., "Aristotelian dynamics in the 2nd century school debates: Galen and Alexander of Aphrodisias on organic powers and movements", in P. ADAMSON; H. BALTUSSEN and M.W.F. STONE (eds.), *Philosophy, science and exegesis in Greek, Arabic and Latin commentaries*, pp. 71-95, London.

LEDERMANN, F., "Andromachus, Galen, Dalibour, Sydenham...: eponyms, as witnesses of a history of the respective galenicals", *J Pharm Belg*. 59.4, pp. 111-119.

LEHOUX, D., "Impersonal and intransitive ἐπισημαίνει", *CPh* 99.1, pp. 78-85.

LÓPEZ FÉREZ, J.A., "Los dioses griegos y sus mitos en Galeno", *CFC(G)* 14, pp. 155-181.

LORUSSO, V., "Il trattato pseudogalenico «*De urinis*» del Parisin. suppl. gr. 634 Fascicule", *BollClass* 25, pp. 5-43.

MALATESTA, M., "Logic and medicine: on «*Institutio logica*» by Galen", *Metalogicon* 17.1, pp. 1-24.

MANSKE, P., "Galen and tendon surgery", *J Hand Surg Am*. 29.4, pp. 547-550.

MURANO, G., "Opere di Galeno nella facoltà di medicina di Bologna", *IMU* 45, pp. 137-165.

NUTTON, V., *Ancient Medicine*. London.

PAPAVRAMIDOU, N.S.; PAPAVRAMIDIS, S.T. and CHRISTOPOULOU-ALETRA, H., "Galen on obesity: etiology, effects, and treatment", *World J Surg*. 28.6, pp. 631-635.

PERILLI, L., *Menodoto di Nicomedia: contributo a una storia galeniana della medicina empirica: con una raccolta commentata delle testimonianze*. Munich.

PINO CAMPOS, L.M., "La doctrina de los pulsos de Galeno en el siglo XVIII: el ejemplo de Francisco Solano de Luque", *CFC(G)* 14, pp. 267-284.

RETIEF, F. and CILLIERS, L., "Malaria in Graeco-Roman times", *AClass* 47, pp. 127-137.

ROSELLI, A., "Galen and the ambiguity of written language: the «*De captionibus*» and the «*Commentaries on Hippocrates*»", in R. PETRILLI and D. GAMBARARA (eds.), *Actualité des anciens sur la théorie du langage*, pp. 51-63, Münster.

SERIO, A., "Il nosos erotico tra letteratura e medicina: il caso di Galeno", *Annali della Facoltá di Lettere e Filosofia. Studi classici 1* , pp. 79-102.

STEGER, F., "Antike Diätetik: Lebensweise und Medizin", *NTM* 12.3, pp. 146-160.

STRANGE, S. K., "The Stoics on the voluntariness of the passions", in S.K. STRANGE, S.K. and J. ZUPKO (eds.), *Stoicism: traditions and transformations*, pp. 32-51, Cambridge.

STROHMAIER, G., "Galen's not uncritical commentary on Hippocrates' "Airs, waters, places"", en P. ADAMSON; H. BALTUSSEN and M.W.F. STONE (eds.), *Philosophy, science and exegesis in Greek, Arabic and Latin commentaries*, pp. 1-9, London.

USTUN, C., "Galen and his anatomic eponym: vein of Galen", *Clin Anat.* 17.6, pp. 454-457.

VIALE, G.L., "The spinal cord and its roots according to Galen", *Neurosurgery* 54.6, pp. 1490-1496.

VON STADEN, H., "Galen's Alexandria", in W. V. HARRIS and G. RUFFINI (eds.), *Ancient Alexandria between Egypt and Greece*, pp. 179-215, Leiden.

VONS, J., "André Vésale et la traité «*De ossibus*» de Galien traduit par F. Balamius", in V. BOUDON-MILLOT and G. COBOLET (eds.), *Lire les médecins grecs à la Renaissance*, pp. 271-282, Paris.

XARCHAS, K.C. and TSOLAKIDIS, G.F., "Galen: author of the first flatfoot description", *J Am Podiatr Med Assoc.* 94.5, pp. 508-509.

2003

BARNES, J., "Proofs and syllogisms in Galen", in J. BARNES and J. JOUANNA (eds.), *Galien et la philosophie*, pp. 1-24, Vandœuvres-Geneve.

BARNES, J. and JOUANNA, J. (eds.), *Galien et la philosophie*. Vandœuvres-Geneve.

BOUDON-MILLOT, V., "Art, science et conjecture chez Galien", in J. BARNES and J. JOUANNA (eds.), *Galien et la philosophie*, pp. 269-298, Vandœuvres-Geneve.

CILLIERS, L. and RETIEF, F. P., "Galenus: prins of pronker?", *Akroterion* 48, pp. 81-88.

DEBRU, A., “L’animalité des parties du corps chez Galien”, in N. PALMIERI (ed.), *Rationnel et irrationnel dans la médecine ancienne et médiévale: aspects historiques, scientifiques et culturels*, pp. 99-110, Saint-Étienne.

DUNN, P.M., “Galen (AD 129-200) of Pergamun: anatomist and experimental physiologist”, *Arch Dis Child Fetal Neonatal Ed.* 88.5, pp. 441-443.

FABRE, A., “Use of Ancient texts in modern therapeutic research”, *Rev Hist Pharm* 51, pp. 239-250.

FISCHER, K.-D., “Der pseudogalenische «*Liber tertius*»”, in I. GAROFALO and A. ROSELLI (eds.), *Galenismo e medicina tardoantica: fonti greche, latine e arabe*, pp. 101-132, Naples.

FORTUNA, S., “Cura degli altri e cura di sé nella medicina antica”, in G. GALLI (ed.), *Interpretazione e cura*, pp. 77-89, Pisa-Rome.

— “La deontologia nel mondo antico”, *Lettere dalla Facoltà, Bollettino della facoltà di Medicina e Chirurgia dell’Università di Ancona* 6.2, pp. 19-22.

FRANZIN-GARREC, M., “Cardiology according to Galen”, *Soins* 1.1, pp. 25-26.

FREDE, M., “Galen’s theology”, in J. BARNES and J. JOUANNA (eds.), *Galien et la philosophie*, pp. 73-126, Vandœuvres-Geneve.

GARCÍA SOLA, Mª.C., “El médico en la Antigüedad clásica”, in A. POCIÑA and J.Mª. GARCÍA GONZÁLEZ (eds.), *En Grecia y Roma: las gentes y sus cosas*, pp. 119-141, Granada.

GAROFALO, I. and ROSELLI, A. (eds.), *Galenismo e medicina tardoantica: fonti greche, latine e arabe*. Naples.

GAROFALO, I., “I sommari degli Alessandrini”, in I. GAROFALO and A. ROSELLI (eds.), *Galenismo e medicina tardoantica: fonti greche, latine e arabe*, pp. 203-231, Naples.

— “Note sui giorni critici in Galeno”, in N. PALMIERI (ed.), *Rationnel et irrationnel dans la médecine ancienne et médiévale: aspects historiques, scientifiques et culturels*, pp. 45-58, Saint-Étienne.

GROß, D. and REININGER, M. (eds.), *Medizin in Geschicte, Philologie und Ethnologie*. Würzburg.

GUERRINI, A., *Experimenting with humans and animals: from Galen to animal rights*. Baltimore.

HANKINSON, R.J., “Causation in Galen”, in J. BARNES and J. JOUANNA (eds.), *Galien et la philosophie*, pp. 31-66, Vandœuvres-Geneve.

HANSON, A.E., "«Your mother nursed you with bile»: anger in babies and small children", *YClS* 32, pp. 185-207.

HOUSTON, G. W., "Galen, his books, and the «*Horrea Piperataria*» at Rome", *MAAR* 48, pp. 45-51.

IRVINE, J.T. and TEMKIN, O., "Who was Akilaos?: a problem in medical historiography", *BHM* 77.1, pp. 12-24.

JACQUART, D., "Avicenne et le galénisme", in I. GAROFALO and A. ROSELLI (eds.), *Galenismo e medicina tardoantica: fonti greche, latine e arabe*, pp. 265-282, Naples.

JOUANNA, J., "La notion de nature chez Galien", in J. BARNES and J. JOUANNA (eds.), *Galien et la philosophie*, pp. 229-262, Vandœuvres-Geneve.

KEIL, G., "Physis: Aspekte des antiken Naturbegriffs", in P. DILG (ed.), *Natur im Mittelalter: Konzeptionen, Erfahrungen, Wirkungen*, pp. 3-29, Berlin.

KOVACIC, F., "Die Natur als Künstler und Baumeister bei Galen", *Traditio* 58, pp. 1-57.

LEE, H. M., "Galen, Johann Heinrich Krause, and the Olympic myth of Greek amateur athletics", *Stadion* 29, pp. 11-20.

LÓPEZ FÉREZ, J.A., "Mitos y personajes míticos en Galeno", in J.A. LÓPEZ FÉREZ (ed.), *Mitos en la literatura griega helenística e imperial*, pp. 403-474, Madrid.

MAGDELAINE, C., "Vieillesse et médecine chez les médecins grecs, d'Hippocrate à Galien", in B. BAKHOUCHE (ed.), *L'ancienneté chez les Anciens*, pp. 61-81, Montpellier.

MANETTI, D., "Galeno, la lingua di Ippocrate e il tempo", in J. BARNES and J. JOUANNA (eds.), *Galien et la philosophie*, pp. 171-220, Vandœuvres-Geneve.

MORTON BRAUND, S. and MOST, G. (eds.), *Ancient anger: perspectives from Homer to Galen*, Cambridge.

NIETO IBÁÑEZ, J.Mª., "Galen's treatise «Thrasybulus» and the dispute between «paidotribes» and «gymnastes»", *Nikephoros* 16, pp. 147-156.

NUTTON, V., "A fragmentary manuscript of Galen's Commentary on Hippocrates'Aphorisms", in A. GARZYA and J. JOUANNA, J. (eds.), *Trasmissione e Ecdotica dei Testi medici greci*, pp. 385-400, Naples.

— "A translation of Galen's *De substantia virtutum naturalium* by Niccolò da Reggio", in D. GROßß and M. REININGER (eds.), *Medizin in Geschichte, Philologie und Ethnologie. Festschrift für Gundolf Keil*, pp. 321-331, Würzburg.

PALMIERI, N., "Fonti galeniche (e non) nella lettura alessandrina dell' «*Ars medica*»", in I. GAROFALO and A. ROSELLI (ed.), *Galenismo e medicina tardoantica: fonti greche, latine e arabe*, pp. 133-160, Naples.

— (ed.), *Rationnel et irrationnel dans la médecine ancienne et médiévale: aspects historiques, scientifiques et culturels*. Saint-Étienne.

PERILLI, L., "Note critico-testuali alla nuova edizione del cosiddetto «testamento filosofico» di Galeno: («*De propriis placitis*», CMG V 3, 2 ed. V. Nutton)", *BollClass* 24, pp. 69-86.

PORMANN, P.E., "Jean le Grammairien et le «*De sectis*» dans la littérature médicale d'Alexandrie", in I. GAROFALO and A. ROSELLI (ed.), *Galenismo e medicina tardoantica: fonti greche, latine e arabe*, pp. 233-263, Naples.

RAMELLI, I., "Galeno e i cristiani: una messa a punto", *InvLuc* 25, pp. 199-219.

ROCCA, J., *Galen on the brain: anatomical knowledge and physiological speculation in the second Century AD*. Leiden.

— "Galen on the brain: anatomical knowledge and physiological speculation in the second century AD", *Stud Anc Med.* 26.1, p. 313.

ROUSSEL, F., *Nature et nature de l'homme chez Galien: physique et physiologie*. Lille.

SAMANA, E., *Les médecins dans le monde grec. Sources épigraphiques sur la naissance d'un corps médical*. Paris.

SCHLANGE-SCHÖNINGEN, H., *Die römische Gesellschaft bei Galen: Biographie und Sozialgeschichte*. Berlin.

SORABJI, R., "The mind-body relation in the wake of Plato's «*Timaeus*»", in G. REYDAM-SCHILS (ed.), *Plato's «Timaeus» as cultural icon*, pp. 152-162, Notre-Dame –Ind.

STROHMAIER, G., "Die Ethik Galens und ihre Rezeption in der Welt Islams", in J. BARNES and J. JOUANNA (eds.), *Galien et la philosophie*, pp. 327-329, Vandœuvres-Geneve.

TIELEMAN, T., "Galen's psychology", in J. BARNES and J. JOUANNA (eds.), *Galien et la philosophie*, pp. 131-161, Vandœuvres-Geneve.

VIALE, G.L., "Return to Galen", *Neurosurgery* 53.1, pp. 205-210.

VON STADEN, H., "Galen's daimon: reflections on "irrational" and "rational"", in N. PALMIERI (ed.), *Rationnel et irrationnel dans la médecine ancienne et médiévale: aspects historiques, scientifiques et culturels*, pp. 15-43, Saint-Étienne.

WILKINS, J., "Land and sea: Italy and the Mediterranean in the Roman discourse of dining", *AJPh* 124.3, pp. 359-375.

XARCHAS, K.C., "Galen on the anatomy and treatment of the injured hand", *Clin Anat.* 16.2, pp. 105-107.

XARCHAS, K.C. and BOURANDAS, J., "Injuries and diseases of the spine in the ancient times", *Spine* 28.13, pp. 1481-1484.

YEO, I.S., "The concept of disease in Galen", *Uisahak* 12.1, pp. 54-65.

ZIPSER, B., "Galens «*De anatomicis administrationibus*» und der Par. Gr. 2203", *Phaos* 3, pp. 147-153.

ZÚÑIGA, J.M., "Galen moves forward", IAPAC 9 (9), pp. 202-203.

2002

ANDROUTSOS, G., "Galen (121-201) and the first experimental test of ureteral function", *Prog Urol.* 12.6, pp. 1341-1345.

APUZZO, M.L. et al., "Honored guest presentation: the legacy of Galen of Pergamon. The neurosurgeon in the arena of sport", *Clin Neurosurg.* 49, pp. 333-370.

BARNES, J., "Galen, Christians, logic", in T.P. WISEMAN (ed.), *Classics in progress: essays on ancient Greece and Rome*, pp. 399-419, Oxford.

BERRYMAN, S.A., "Galen and the mechanical philosophy", *Apeiron* 35.3, pp. 235-253.

BOBZIEN, S., "Pre-Stoic hypothetical syllogistic in Galen's «*Institutio logica*»", in V. NUTTON (ed.), *The unknown Galen*, pp. 57-72, London.

BOS, G., "The reception of Galen in Maimonides' «*Medical aphorisms*»", in V. NUTTON (ed.), *The unknown Galen*, pp. 139-152, London.

BOUDON-MILLOT, V., "Galen's «*On my own books*»: new material from Meshed, Rida, tibb. 5223", in V. NUTTON (ed.), *The unknown Galen*, pp. 9-18, London.

— "La thériaque selon Galien: poison salutaire ou remède empoisonné?", in F. COLLARD and E. SAMANA (eds.), *Le corps à l'épreuve*, pp. 45-56, Langres.

— "Un médecin oenophile: Galien et le vin de Falerne", in J. JOUANNA; L. VILLARD and D. BÉGUIN (eds.), *Vin et santé en Grèce ancienne*, pp. 78-93, Paris.

— *Galien, le vrai père de la médecine*. Paris.

CAPRIGLIONE, J. C., "Temi di astrologia in Galeno", in A. PÉREZ JIMÉNEZ and R. CABALLERO (eds.), *«Homo mathematicus»: actas del congreso internacional sobre astrólogos griegos y romanos*, pp. 259-274, Malaga.

CAVALLO, G., "Galeno e la levatrice: qualche riflessione su libri e sapere medico nel mondo antico", *MedSec* 14.2, pp. 407-416.

COURTEMANCHE, A., "Abulcasis, Avicenna, and Galen: a forensic investigation by a 14th century Jewish physician", *Can Bull Med Hist*. 19.2, pp. 441-453.

DEBRU, A., "Galen "*On the unclear movements*"", in V. NUTTON (ed.), *The unknown Galen*, pp. 79-85, London.

DEMAITRE, L., "Straws in the wind: Latin writings on asthma between Galen and Cardano", *Allergy Asthma Proc*. 23.1, pp. 61-93.

FICHTNER, G., *Corpus Galenicum: verzeichnis der galenischen und pseudogalenischen schriften*. Tübingen.

FLEMMING, R., "The pathology of pregnancy in Galen's commentaries on the «*Epidemics*»", in V. NUTTON (ed.), *The unknown Galen*, pp. 101-112, London.

GARCÍA BALLESTER, L., *Galen and Galenism: theory and medical practice from antiquity to the European renaissance*. Farnham.

GARCÍA SOLA, Mª.C., "Influencia de los astros en la resolución de las crisis en el tratado de Galeno "*Sobre los días críticos*"", in J. PELÁEZ (ed.), *El dios que hechiza y encanta: magia y astrología en el mundo clásico y helenístico*, pp. 275-283, Cordoba.

GAROFALO, I., "L'ecdotique des textes médicaux grecs: tradition et ecdotique", *LIMAM* 1, pp. 24-27.

— "Alcune questioni sulle fonti greche del «*Continens*» di Razes", *MedSec* 14.2, pp. 386-406.

— "Problemi di lessico anatomico", *Fontes* 7-10, pp. 59-67.

GELLER, M.J., "Hippocrates, Galen and the Jews: renal medicine in the Talmud", *Am J Nephrol* 22.2-3, pp. 101-106.

LAUTNER, P., "Andronicus of Rhodes on Aristotle's *Physics* 202a13-21, b23-30", *AAntHung* 42.1-4, pp. 125-132.

McVAUGH, M., "The lost Latin Galen", in V. NUTTON (ed.), *The unknown Galen*, pp. 153-164, London.

MÜLLER, I., "Hugo de Folieto: «*De medicina animae*» : antike Humoralpathologie in christlicher Deutung", in C. SCHULZE and S. IHM (eds.), *Ärztekunst und Gottvertrauen: antike und mittelalterliche Schnittpunkte von Christentum und Medizin*, pp. 71-89, Hildesheim-New York.

NICKEL, D., "On the authenticity of an «excerpt» from Galen's «*Commentary on the Timaeus*»", in V. NUTTON (ed.), *The unknown Galen*, pp. 73-78, London.

NUTTON, V. (ed.), *The unknown Galen*. London.

— "In defence of Kühn", in V. NUTTON (ed.), *The unknown Galen*, pp. 1-7, London.

— "Portraits of science. Logic, learning, and experimental medicine", *Science* 295 (nº 5556), pp. 800-801.

— "Ancient medicine: Aesclepius transformed", in C. TUPLIN and T.E. RIHLL (eds.), *Science and mathematics in ancient Greek culture*, pp. 242-255, Oxford.

— "The diffusion of ancient medicine in the Renaissance", *Medicina nei Secoli. Arte e Scienza* 142, pp. 461-478.

PESENTI, T., "Le «*Divisiones librorum Ypocratis*» nei commenti all' «*Articella*»", *MedSec* 14.2, pp. 417-437.

PINO CAMPOS, L.M., "El término "pulso" en Grecia", *Fortunatae* 13, pp. 233-254.

ROCCA, J., "The brain beyond Kühn: reflections on «*Anatomical procedures*», Book IX", in V. NUTTON (ed.), *The unknown Galen*, pp. 87-100, London.

ROSELLI, A., "Dalla δικαίη φύσις dei trattati chirurgici alla δικαιοσύνη τῆς φύσεως di Galeno", in A. THIVEL and A. ZUCKER (eds.), *Le normal et le pathologique dans la collection hippocratique: actes du Xème colloque international hippocratique*, pp. 731-752, Paris.

— "Ἐκ βιβλίου κυβερνήτης: i limiti dell'apprendimento dai libri nella formazione tecnica e filosofica (Galeno, Polibio, Filodemo)", *Vichiana* 4.1, pp. 35-50.

SALLAM, H.N., "The ancient Alexandria school of medicine", *Gynecol Obstet Fertil.* 30.1, pp. 3-10.

SAVAGE-SMITH, E., "Galen's lost ophthalmology and the «*Summaria Alexandrinorum*»", in V. NUTTON (ed.), *The unknown Galen*, pp. 121-138, London.

STROHMAIER, G., "The uses of Galen in Arabic literature", in V. NUTTON (ed.), *The unknown Galen*, pp. 113-120, London.

TAN, S.Y., "Galen (130-201 A.D.): history's most enduring medic", *Singapore Med J.* 43.3, pp. 116-117.

TIELEMAN, T., "Galen on the seat of the intellect: anatomical experiment and philosophical tradition", in C. TUPLIN and T.E. RIHLL (eds.), *Science and mathematics in ancient Greek culture*, pp. 256-273, Oxford.

TOLEDO-PEREYRA, L.H., "Claudius Galenus of Pergamum: surgeon of gladiators. Father of experimental physiology", *J Invest Surg.* 15.6, pp. 299-301.

TUPLIN, C. and RIHLL, T.E. (eds.), *Science and mathematics in ancient Greek culture*. Oxford.

VON STADEN, H., "Division, dissection, and specialization: Galen's «On the parts of the medical techne»", in V. NUTTON (ed.), *The unknown Galen*, pp. 19-45, London.

WILKINS, J., "The contribution of Galen, «*De subtiliante diaeta* (On the thinning diet)»", in V. NUTTON (ed.), *The unknown Galen*, pp. 47-55, London.

2001

AGUILAR, R.Mª., "La prevención de la salud en la Antigüedad: Plutarco y Galeno", in A. PÉREZ JIMÉNEZ and F. CASADESÚS BORDOY (eds.), *Estudios sobre Plutarco: misticismo y religiones mistéricas en la obra de Plutarco*, pp. 461-471, Madrid.

ALLEN, J., "Galen as (mis)informant about the views of his predecessors: a discussion of R. J. Hankinson (ed.), *Galen on antecedent causes* (Cambridge, 1998)", *AGPh* 83.1, pp. 81-89.

BACALEXI, D., "*De pulsibus ad tirones*: Galen and new physicians: the pulse as a means of diagnosis and prognosis", *Bulletin de l'Association Guillaume Budé* 2, pp. 131-152.

BAZOU, A., *L' influence du traité de Galien ["Oti tais tou sômatos krasesin ai tès psuchès dynameis epontai": "Que les facultés de l'âme suivent les tempéraments du corps"] aux écrivains postérieurs*. Athens.

BONNET-CADILHAC, C., "L'anatomo-physiologie de l'appareil genital mâle chez Galien", *MedSec* 13.2, pp. 349-372.

BOUDON-MILLOT, V., "Galien face à la peste antonine ou comment penser l' invisible?", in S. BAZIN-TACCHELLA; D. QUÉRUEL and E. SAMAMA (eds.), *Air, miasme et contagion. Les épidémies dans l'Antiquité et au Moyen Âge*, pp. 29-54, Langres.

BOULOGNE, J., "Medical myths and notions in Ancient Greece", *Med Nowozytna* 8.2, pp. 33-52.

BRODERSEN, K., "The presentation of geographical knowledge for travel and transport in the Roman world: «*itineraria non tantum adnotata sed etiam picta*»", in C. ADAMS and R. LAURENCE (eds.), *Travel and Geography in the Roman Empire*, pp. 7-21, London.

DEBRU, A. and PALMIERI, N. (eds.), *«Docente natura»: mélanges de médecine ancienne et médiévale offerts à Guy Sabbah*. Saint-Étienne.

DIAMANDOPOULOS, A.A.; GOUDAS, P. and DIAMANDOPOULOS, A.H., "The human skin: a meeting ground for the ideas about macrocosm and microcosm in ancient and Medieval and Greek literature", *Vesalius* 7.2, pp. 94-101.

FORTUNA, S., "Il metodo della diagnosi in Galeno: («*De locis affectis*», VIII 1-452 K.)", *Elenchos* 22.2, pp. 281-304.

— "Sulla tradizione e sul testo del «*Commento*» di Galeno al «*Prognostico*» di Ippocrate", *AION(filol)* 23, pp. 233-249.

FORTUNA, S. and GOUREVITCH, D., "Galeno e le edizioni del cinquecento e del seicento nelle biblioteche marchigiane", in A. SERRANI (ed.), *Medici e scienziati, artisti e letterati nelle marche del seicento*, pp. 123-139, Fermo.

GAROFALO, I., "Note e emendamenti ai commenti alessandrini a Ippocrate e Galeno", in A. DEBRU and N. PALMIERI (eds.), *«Docente natura»: mélanges de médecine ancienne et médiévale offerts à Guy Sabbah*, pp. 112-131, Saint-Étienne.

— "Postilla a «Una nuova opera di Galeno»", *SCO* 47.3, pp. 583-586.

— "Problemi di lessico anatomico", *Fontes* 4-5 pp. 59-67.

GÓMEZ, A., "Galenic concepts", *Rev Med Chil.* 129.3, pp. 327-329.

GOUREVITCH, D., *I giovani pazienti di Galeno: per una patocenosi dell'Impero Romano*. Rome.

— "Sur l'andrologie pathologique de Galien", *MedSec* 13.2, pp. 333-347.

— "Two states in the history of the concept of contagion: from Hippocrates to Galen", *Bull Acad Natl Med.* 185.5, pp. 977-986.

— "Un éléphant peut en cacher un autre ou Comment sauter du coq à l'âne peut mettre la puce à l'oreille", in A. DEBRU and N. PALMIERI (eds.), «*Docente natura*»: *mélanges de médecine ancienne et médiévale offerts à Guy Sabbah*, pp. 156-176, Saint-Étienne.

— "Claude Bernard lecteur de Galien?", in A. GARZYA and J. JOUANNA (eds.), *Transmission et ecdotique des textes médicaux grecs. Actes du IVe colloque international*, pp. 173-185, Naples.

— "Le nourrisson et sa nourrice: étude de quelques cas pédiatriques chez Galien", *RPhA* 2, pp. 63-76.

HOLOWCHAK, M.A., "Interpreting dreams for corrective regimen: diagnostic dreams in Greco-Roman medicine", *JHM* 56.4, pp. 382-399.

KOVACIC, F., *Der Begriff der Physis bei Galen vor dem Hintergrund seiner Vorgänger*. Stuttgart.

LEWIS, E.J., "The treatment of lupus nephritis: revisiting Galen", *Ann Intern Med.* 135.4, pp. 296-298.

MALATESTA, M., "Polyadic inclusive disjunctive syllogism in Galen's «*Institutio logica*»", *Metalogicon* 14.1, pp. 1-8.

MANZONI, T., *Il cervello secondo Galeno*. Ancona.

MICUNCO, G., "Il mito di Ippocrate", *InvLuc* 23, pp. 147-159.

NUTTON, V., "Luis García Ballester and Galen", *Dynamis* 21, pp. 457-464.

— "God, Galen and the Depaganization of Ancient medicine", in P. BILLER and J. ZIEGLER (eds.), *Religion and Medicine in the Middle Ages*, pp. 15-32, York.

PAHTA, P., "Medieval andrology and the pseudo-galenic *De spermate*", *MedSec* 13.3, pp. 509-521.

PALMIERI, N., "Nouvelles remarques sur les commentaires à Galien de l'école médicale de Ravenne", in A. DEBRU and N. PALMIERI (eds.), «*Docente natura*»: *mélanges de médecine ancienne et médiévale offerts à Guy Sabbah*, pp. 209-246, Saint-Étienne.

PAWELETZ, N., "From Galen to Golgi: birth of the life sciences in Italy", *Nat Rev Mol Cell Biol.* 2.6, pp. 475-480.

PERILLI, L., "Menodoto di Nicomedia e i principi della medicina empirica", in A. BRANCACCI (ed.), *Antichi e moderni nella filosofia di età imperiale*, pp. 267-297, Naples.

PESENTI, T., "The «*Libri Galieni*» in Italian universities in the fourteenth century", *IMU* 42, pp. 119-147.

RODRÍGUEZ ALFAGEME, I., "El campo semántico de los nombres del habla en Galeno", *CFC(G)* 11, pp. 139-178.

STEEL, C., "The moral purpose of the human body: a reading of *Timaeus* 69-72", *Phronesis* 46.2, pp. 105-128.

STERNBACH, G.L. et al., "Galen and the origins of artificial ventilation, the arteries and the pulse", *Resuscitation* 49.2, pp. 119-122.

VEGETTI, M., "Il confronto degli antichi e dei moderni in Galeno", in G. CAJANI and D. LANZA (eds.), *L'antico degli antichi*, pp. 87-100, Palermo.

VIALE, G.L. et al, "The subchoroidal approach to the third ventricle: surgical anatomy according to Galen", *Neurosurgery* 49.4, pp. 986-990.

2000

APUZZO, M.L., "The legacy of Galen of Pergamon", *Neurosurgery* 47.3, p. 545.

BOSCHERINI, S., "La dottrina medica comunicata «*per epistulam*»: struttura e storia di un genere", in A. PIGEAUD and J. PIGEAUD (eds.), *Les textes médicaux latins comme littérature*, pp. 1-11, Nantes.

BOUDON-MILLOT, V., "Galien par lui-même: les traités bio-bibliographiques: («*De ordine librorum suorum*» et «*De libris propriis*»)", in D. MANETTI (ed.), *Studi su Galeno: scienza, filosofia, retorica e filologia*, pp. 119-133, Florence.

BRANCACCI, A. (ed.), *La filosofia in età imperiale: le scuole e le tradizioni filosofiche*. Naples.

CALABI, F., "Galeno e Mosè", *RSF* 55.4, pp. 535-546.

CAMBIANO, G., "Galeno, Erasistrato e la teleologia di Aristotele", in D. MANETTI (ed.), *Studi su Galeno: scienza, filosofia, retorica e filologia*, pp. 45-57, Florence.

CAPRIGLIONE, J.C., "La «*diaita*» secondo Galeno", *CFC(G)* 10, pp. 155-172.

CONNELL, S.M., "Aristotle and Galen on sex difference and reproduction: a new approach to an ancient rivalry", *SHPS* 31.3, pp. 405-427.

CORNEJO, R. and O'LEARY, J.P., "Galen's life and contributions", *Am Surg*. 66 .8, pp. 608-609.

DESIDERI, P., "Galeno come intellettuale", in D. MANETTI (ed.), *Studi su Galeno: scienza, filosofia, retorica e filologia*, pp. 13-29, Florence.

FLEMMING, R., *Medicine and the making of Roman women: gender, nature, and authority from Celsus to Galen*. Oxford.

FORTUNA, S. and ORILIA, F., "Diagnosi, abduzione e metafora del testo: aspetti storici e metodologici", in G. GALLI (ed.), *Interpretazioni e diagnosi*, pp. 101-121, Dordrecht.

GAROFALO, I., "Il «*Sunto*» di Ioannes Grammatikos delle opere del Canone di Galeno", in D. MANETTI (ed.), *Studi su Galeno: scienza, filosofia, retorica e filologia*, pp. 135-151, Florence.

GARCÍA BALLESTER, L., "Galenism and medical teaching at the University of Salamanca during the fifteenth century", *Dynamis* 20, pp. 209-247.

GRANT, M., "Dietetic responses in Galen to madness", *CB* 76.1, pp. 61-70.

JOUANNA, J., "Miasme, maladie et semence de la maladie: Galien lecteur d'Hippocrate", in D. MANETTI (ed.), *Studi su Galeno: scienza, filosofia, retorica e filologia*, pp. 59-62, Florence.

LONGO, O., "La mano dell'uomo da Aristotele a Galeno", *Quaderni urbinati di cultura classica* 66, pp. 7-30.

LÓPEZ FÉREZ, J.A. (ed.), *La lengua científica griega: orígenes, desarrollo e influencia en las lenguas modernas europeas*. Madrid.

MAKSIMOVIĆ, J., "In memory of Galen -on the 1800th anniversary of his death", *Med Pregl*. 53, pp. 313-317.

MANETTI, D., "Galeno tra autodefinizione e ricezione", in D. MANETTI (ed.), *Studi su Galeno: scienza, filosofia, retorica e filologia*, pp. 7-12, Florence.

— (ed.), *Studi su Galeno: scienza, filosofia, retorica e filologia*. Florence.

MARTORELLI VICO, R., "La medicina scolastica tra galenismo e aristotelismo", *StudMed* 41.1, pp. 311-338.

MASULLO, R., "Tradition and innovation in late antique therapeutics: the case of Philagrius", *Koinonia* 24.2, pp. 231-243.

MAZZINI, I., "Presenza e funzione della lingua e della letteratura poetiche profane in alcune opere mediche in versi del mondo antico", in A. PIGEAUD and J. PIGEAUD (eds.), *Les textes médicaux latins comme littérature*, pp. 173-185, Nantes.

NUTTON, V., "Did the Greeks have a word for it? Contagion and Contagion Theory in Classical Antiquity", in L.I. CONRAD and D. WUJASTYK (eds.), *Contagion.* Perspectives from pre-modern societies, pp. 137-162, Aldershot.

— "Medical thoughts on urban Pollution", in V.M. HOPE and E. MARSHALL (eds.), *Death and disease in the Ancient city*, pp. 65-73, London.

— "Medicine", in A.K. BOWMAN; P.D. GARNSEY and D. RATHBONE (eds.), *The Cambridge Ancient History, Vol. XI, The High Empire, A.D. 70-192*, pp. 943-968, Cambridge.

PALMIERI, N. "Rhétorique et pédagogie dans les commentaires à Galien d'Agnellus de Ravenne", in A. PIGEAUD and J. PIGEAUD (eds.), *Les textes médicaux latins comme littérature*, pp. 221-239, Nantes.

PERILLI, L., "L'ordinamento alfabetico di lessici e glossari: il caso del «*Glossario ippocratico*» di Galeno", *BBGG* 54, pp. 27-52.

— "La fortuna di Galeno filosofo: un nuovo testimone dei commentari neoplatonici (Scholia Yalensia) al «*De elementis*»", in A. BRANCACCI (ed.), *La filosofia in età imperiale: le scuole e le tradizioni filosofiche*, pp. 85-135, Naples.

PIGEAUD, A. and PIGEAUD, J. (eds.), *Les textes médicaux latins comme littérature*. Nantes.

PIGEAUD, J., "Les textes médicaux comme literature", in A. PIGEAUD and PIGEAUD (eds.), *Les textes médicaux latins comme littérature*, pp. 377-389, Nantes.

ROMANO, E., "La dietetica di Galeno: un incontro fra medicina e politica", in D. MANETTI (ed.), *Studi su Galeno: scienza, filosofia, retorica e filologia*, pp. 31-44, Florence.

ROSELLI, A., "Il commento di Galeno a «*Sulle fratture*»: specimina per la nuova edizione", in D. MANETTI (ed.), *Studi su Galeno: scienza, filosofia, retorica e filologia*, pp. 93-117, Florence.

SERIO, A., "Il νόσος erotico tra letteratura e medicina: il caso di Galeno", *AFLPer(class)* 20, pp. 79-102.

SIMÓN PALMER, Mª.C., "Hipócrates y Galeno en el teatro español del Siglo de Oro", in V.V.A.A., *Tes philies tade dora: miscelánea léxica en memoria de Conchita Serrano*, pp. 523-534, Madrid.

STREPPEL, M.; HEISER, T. and STENNERT, E., "Historical development of facial nerve surgery with special reference to hypoglossal-facial nerve anastomosis", *HNO* 48, pp. 801-808.

TONI, R., "Ancient views on the hypothalamic-pituitary-thyroid axis: an historical and epistemological perspective", *Pituitary* 3.2, pp. 83-95.

URSCHEL, H.C., "The history of surgery for thoracic outlet syndrome", *Chest Surg Clin N Am.* 10.1, pp. 183-188.

VEGETTI, M., "«*De caelo in terram*»: il «*Timeo*» in Galeno («*De placitis*», «*Quod animi*»)", in A. BRANCACCI (ed.), *La filosofia in età imperiale: le scuole e le tradizioni filosofiche*, pp. 69-84, Naples.

VOLPE CACCIATORE, P., "El régimen según Galeno", in A. PÉREZ JIMÉNEZ and G. CRUZ ANDREOTTI (eds.), *Dieta mediterránea: comidas y hábitos alimenticios en las culturas mediterráneas*, pp. 91-101, Madrid.

VON STADEN, H., "Body, soul, and nerves: Epicurus, Herophilus, Erasistratus, the Stoics, and Galen", in J.P. WRIGHT and P. POTTER (eds.), *Psyche and soma: physicians and metaphysicians on the mind-body problem from Antiquity to Enlightenment*, pp. 79-116, Oxford.

YANNATOS, D.; HESHIKI, R.E. and HERAULT, C., "Notes on voice and speech disorders in ancient and Byzantine Greece", *Rev Laryngol Otol Rhinol.* 121, pp. 329-331.

ZONTA, M., "La ricerca sulle fonti antiche della letteratura filosofica araba ed ebraica: a proposito di un libro recente", *Athenaeum* 88.2, pp. 597-604.

1999

ALBI ROMERO, G., "Andrés Laguna y el libro "*De urinis*" de Galeno", in J.L. GARCÍA HOURCADE and J.M. MORENO YUSTE (eds.), *Andrés Laguna: humanismo, ciencia y política en la Europa renacentista*, pp. 419-426, Valladolid.

ÁLVAREZ MILLÁN, C., "Graeco-Roman case histories and their influence on Medieval Islamic clinical accounts", *Soc Hist Med.* 12.1, pp. 19-43.

BENNETT, M.R., "The early history of the synapse: from Plato to Sherrington", *Brain Res Bull.* 50.2, pp. 95-118.

BERGDOLT, K., "History of medicine and concepts of health", *Croat Med J.* 40.2, pp. 119-122.

BIEN, C. G., "Galen zum Problem der Missbildungen", *Sudhoffs Archiv* 83.1, pp. 67-72.

BLOOM, D.A.; MILEN, M.T. and HEININGER, J.C., "Claudius Galen: from a 20th century genitourinary perspective", *J Urol.* 161.1, pp. 12-19.

CAPRIGLIONE, J.C., "Anatomía y filosofía en Galeno", in A. PÉREZ JIMÉNEZ and G. CRUZ ANDREOTTI (eds.), *Unidad y pluralidad del cuerpo humano: la anatomía en las culturas mediterráneas*, pp. 137-167, Madrid.

CRUSE, J.M., "History of medicine: the metamorphosis of scientific medicine in the ever-present past", *Am J Med Sci.* 318.3, pp. 171-180.

EIJK, P.J. (ed.), *Ancient histories of Medicine: essays in medical Doxography and Historiography in classical Antiquity*. Leiden.

FORTUNA, S., "I «*Procedimenti anatomici*» di Galeno e la traduzione latina di Demetrio Calcondila", *MedSec* 11.1, p. 9-28.

— "Nicolò Leoniceno e la traduzione latina dell' *Ars Medica* di Galeno", in A. GARZYA and J. JOUANNA. (eds.), *I testi medici greci. Tradizione e ecdotica*, pp. 157-173, Naples.

— "Le prime traduzioni umanistiche degli «*Aforismi*» di Ippocrate", in I. GAROFALO et al. (eds.), *Aspetti della terapia nel «Corpus Hippocraticum»*, pp. 485-498, Florence.

GAROFALO, I., "Una nuova opera di Galeno: la «*Synopsis*» del «*De methodo medendi*» in versione araba", *SCO* 47 (1), pp. 9-19.

GAROFALO, I. et al. (eds.), *Aspetti della terapia nel «Corpus Hippocraticum»: atti del IXe colloque international hippocratique*. Florence.

GUARDASOLE, A., "Galeno e i tragici greci", *AAP* 48, pp. 431-449.

LASCARATOS, J. and POULAKOU-REBELAKOU, E., "Hippocrates and Galen", *Scalpel Tongs* 43, pp. 37-38.

LÓPEZ FÉREZ, J.A., "Lectura y comentario de algunos textos de Galeno relacionados con la retórica", in J.A. LÓPEZ FÉREZ (ed.), *Desde los poemas homéricos hasta la prosa griega del siglo IV d.C.: veintiséis estudios filológicos*, pp. 421-445, Madrid.

— "La anatomía en Galeno", in A. PÉREZ JIMÉNEZ and G. CRUZ ANDREOTTI (eds.), *Unidad y pluralidad del cuerpo humano: la anatomía en las culturas mediterráneas*, pp. 95-136, Madrid.

MARKETOS, S.G. and SKIADAS, P.K., "Galen: a pioneer of spine research", *Spine* 24, pp. 2358-2362.

PINTAUDI, R., "Pot-pourri", *APapyrol* 10-11, pp. 131-147.

PROVERBIO, D.V., “Sul più antico codice delle «*Masa'il fi't-tibb lil-Muta'allimin*» di Hunayn ibn Ishaq («*Isagoge Iohannitii*»)”, *RAL* 10.1, pp. 57-92.

RIZK, D.E., “Claudius Galen: from a 20th century genitourinary perspective”, *J Urol.* 162.4, pp. 1392-1393.

ROSELLI, A., “Notes on the doxai of doctors in Galen’s commentaries on Hippocrates”, in P.J. EIJK (ed.), *Ancient histories of Medicine: essays in medical Doxography and Historiography in classical Antiquity*, pp. 359-381, Leiden.

ROUECHÉ, M., “Did medical students study philosophy in Alexandria?”, *BICS* 43, pp. 153-169.

SCHIAPARELLI, A., “L’influenza della «*Retorica*» di Aristotele in età imperiale: l’importanza di essere chiaramente ambigui”, *Méthexis* 12, pp. 53-75.

VALLANCE, J. T., “Galen, Proclus and the non-submissive commentary”, in G.W. MOST (ed.), *Commentaries = Kommentare*, pp. 223-244, Göttingen.

VEGETTI, M., “Tradition and truth: forms of philosophical-scientific historiography in Galen’s «*De placitis*»”, en P.J. EIJK (ed.), *Ancient histories of Medicine: essays in medical Doxography and Historiography in classical Antiquity*, pp. 333-357, Leiden.

— “Historiographical strategies in Galen’s physiology: («*De usu partium*», «*De naturalibus facultatibus*»)”, in P.J. EIJK (ed.), *Ancient histories of Medicine: essays in medical Doxography and Historiography in classical Antiquity*, pp. 383-395, Leiden.

— “Metáforas del cuerpo de Aristóteles a Galeno”, in A. PÉREZ JIMÉNEZ and G. CRUZ ANDREOTTI (eds.), *Unidad y pluralidad del cuerpo humano: la anatomía en las culturas mediterráneas*, pp. 81-94, Madrid.

ZHONG, G. and WAN, F., “An outline on the early pharmacetical development before Galen”, *Zhonghua Yi Shi Za Zhi* 29.3, pp. 178-182.

1998

BAFFIONI, C., “L’embriologia araba fra astrologia e medicina”, in R.B. FINAZZI and A. VALVO (eds.), *La diffusione dell’eredità classica nell’età tardoantica e medievale: il «Romanzo di Alessandro» e altri scritti*, pp. 1-20, Alessandria.

BETT, R., “The Sceptics and the emotions”, in J. SIHVOLA and T. ENGBERG-PEDERSEN (eds.), *The Emotions in Hellenistic philosophy*, pp. 197-218, Dordrecht.

COSANS, C. E., “The experimental foundations of Galen’s teleology”, *SHPS* 29.1, pp. 63-80.

DU BOULAY, G.H.; LAWTON, M. and WALLIS, A., “The story of the internal carotid artery of mammals: from Galen to sudden infant death syndrome”, *Neuroradiology* 40.11, pp. 697-703.

EHMIG, U., "Die Auswirkungen der Pest in antonischer Zeit", *ZPE* 122, pp. 206-207.

EL-GAMMAL, S.Y., "The role of Galen in the development and progress of medical sciences", *Bull Indian Inst Hist Med Hyderabad* 28.2, pp. 119-127.

FERRARI, F., "Galeno interprete del *Timeo*", *MH* 55.1, pp. 14-34.

FISCHER, K.D., NICKEL, D. and POTTER, P. (eds.), *Text and tradition: studies in ancient Medicine and its transmission presented to Jutta Kollesch*. Leiden.

GALUZZI, M.; MICHELI, G. and MONTI, M.T. (eds.), *Le forme della comunicazione scientifica*. Milan.

GARCÍA BALLESTER, L., "The «new Galen»: a challenge to Latin Galenism in thirteenth-century Montpellier", in K.D. FISCHER; D. NICKEL and P. POTTER (eds.), *Text and tradition: studies in ancient Medicine and its transmission presented to Jutta Kollesch*, pp. 55-83, Leiden.

GAROFALO, I. "Le commentaire ravennate au «*De pulsibus ad tirones*» de Galien: le commentaire et ses sources", in C. DEROUX (ed.), *Maladie et maladies dans les textes latins*, pp. 382-392, Brussels.

— "Variazioni stilistiche nell'anatomia di Galeno e del galenismo", in M. GALUZZI; G. MICHELI and M.T. MONTI (eds.), *Le forme della comunicazione scientifica*, pp. 57-68, Milan.

GILL, C., "Did Galen understand Platonic and Stoic thinking on emotions?", in J. SIHVOLA and T. ENGBERG-PEDERSEN (eds.), *The Emotions in Hellenistic philosophy*, pp. 113-148, Dordrecht.

GOUREVITCH, D., "The marriage between the physician and philology", *MedSec* 10.2, pp. 227-239.

HANSON, A.E., "Galen: author and critic", in G.W. MOST (ed.), *Editing texts = Texte edieren*, pp. 22-53, Göttingen.

— "In the shadow of Galen: two Berlin papyri of medical context («BKT» IX 80 and 81)", in K.D. FISCHER; D. NICKEL and P. POTTER (eds.), *Text and tradition: studies in ancient Medicine and its transmission presented to Jutta Kollesch*, pp. 145-159, Leiden.

LATRONICO, N., "Science, customs and social life in the classical world", *Minerva Pediatr.* 50.11, pp. 479-496.

MANETTI, D., "Galeno e il significato di μακρολογία e μικρολογία (In Hipp. Fract. XVIII 2, 518-519 e 526-527 K.)", *RFIC* 126.1, pp. 55-71.

OSER-GROTE, C.M., "Einführung in das Studium der Medizin: eisagogische Schriften des Galen in ihrem Verhältnis zum *Corpus Hippocraticum*", in J. KULLMANN; J.

ALTHOFF and ASPER, M. (eds.), *Gattungen wissenschaftlicher Literatur in der Antike*, pp. 95-117, Tübingen.

PALMIERI, N. "La structure du commentaire ravennate au «*De pulsibus ad tirones*» de Galien", in C. DEROUX (ed.), *Maladie et maladies dans les textes latins*, pp. 393-405, Brussels.

POTTER, P., "The «*editiones principes*» of Galen and Hippocrates and their relationship", in K.D. FISCHER; D. NICKEL and P. POTTER (eds.), *Text and tradition: studies in ancient Medicine and its transmission presented to Jutta Kollesch*, pp. 243-261, Leiden.

SCHWEIKARDT, C., "How do cathartic drugs act? A case study on Gregor Horst (1578-1636) and his attempt to defend Galenist theory", *Vesalius* 4.2, pp. 69-78.

SIHVOLA, J. and ENGBERG-PEDERSEN, T. (eds.), *The Emotions in Hellenistic philosophy*. Dordrecht.

SORABJI, R., "Chrysippus - Posidonius - Seneca: a high-level debate on emotion", in J. SIHVOLA and T. ENGBERG-PEDERSEN (eds.), *The Emotions in Hellenistic philosophy*, pp. 149-169, Dordrecht.

STROHMAIER, G., "Bekannte und unbekannte Zitate in den «*Zweifeln an Galen*» des Rhazes", in K.D. FISCHER; D. NICKEL and P. POTTER (eds.), *Text and tradition: studies in ancient Medicine and its transmission presented to Jutta Kollesch*, pp. 263-287, Leiden.

TIELEMAN, T., "Plotinus on the seat of the soul: reverberations of Galen and Alexander in Enn. IV, 3 [27], 23", *Phronesis* 43.4, pp. 306-325.

VON STADEN, H., "Gattung und Gedächtnis: Galen über Wahrheit und Lehrdichtung", in J. KULLMANN; J. ALTHOFF and M. ASPER (eds.), *Gattungen wissenschaftlicher Literatur in der Antike*, pp. 65-94, Tübingen.

1997

ANASTASSIOU, A. and IRMER, D. (eds.), *Testimonien zum Corpus Hippocraticum. 2, Galen. 1, Hippokrateszitate in den Kommentaren und im Glossar*. Göttingen.

BARNES, J., "Logique et pharmacologie: à propos de quelques remarques d'ordre linguistique dans le «*De simplicium medicamentorum temperamentis ac facultatibus*» de Galien", in A. DEBRU (ed.), *Galen on pharmacology: philosophy, history and medicine*, pp. 3-33, Leiden.

BÉGUIN, D., "Les œuvres pharmacologiques de Galien dans l'enseignement, l'édition et la pratique de la médecine en France au seizième siècle", in A. DEBRU (ed.), *Galen on pharmacology: philosophy, history and medicine*, pp. 283-300, Leiden.

BONNET-CADILHAC, C., *L'anatomo-physiologie de la génération chez Galien*. Unpublished PhD.

BOULOGNE, J., "L'apport de Galien à la méthode médicale", *REG* 110.1, pp. 126-142.

COSANS, C. E., "Galen's critique of rationalist and empiricist anatomy", *JHB* 30.1, pp. 35-54.

EIJK, P. J., "Galen's use of the concept of «qualified experience» in his dietetic and pharmacological works", in A. DEBRU (ed.), *Galen on pharmacology: philosophy, history and medicine*, pp. 35-57, Leiden.

FEDERSPIL, G. and SCANDELLARI, C., "Origins and evolution of experimental medicine", *MedSec* 9.1, pp. 3-21.

FLASHAR, H. and JOUANNA, J. (ed.), *Médecine et morale dans l'Antiquité*. Vandœuvres-Geneve.

FUTRELL, A., *Blood in the Arena. The Spectacle of Roman Power*. Austin.

GIULIANI, Mª.F., "Il «*Glossario ippocratico*» di Galeno", *Rudiae* 9, pp. 95-136.

GOUREVITCH, D., "Galien et la mauvaise malade", *MedSec* 9.2, pp. 249-260.

GRIVETTI, L.E. and APPLEGATE, E.A., "From Olympia to Atlanta: a cultural-historical perspective on diet and athletic training", *J Nutr.* 127, pp. 860-868.

HANKINSON, R.J., "Natural criteria and the transparency of judgement: Antiochus, Philo and Galen on epistemological justification", in B. INWOOD and J. MANSFELD (eds.), *Assent and argument: studies in Cicero's «Academic books»*, pp. 161-216, Leiden.

IHM, S., "Die Quellen der Giftkapitel von Galens «*De antidotis II*»", in A. DEBRU (ed.), *Galen on pharmacology: philosophy, history and medicine*, pp. 235-253, Leiden.

JACQUES, J.-M., "La méthode de Galien pharmacologue dans les deux traités sur les médicaments composés: (Περι συνθέσεως φαρμάκων)", in A. DEBRU (ed.), *Galen on pharmacology: philosophy, history and medicine*, pp. 103-129, Leiden.

JOUANNA, J., "La lecture de l'éthique hippocratique chez Galien", in H. FLASHAR and J. JOUANNA (eds.), *Médecine et morale dans l'Antiquité*, pp. 211-253, Vandeoeuvres-Geneve.

JOUANNA, J. and BOUDON-MILLOT, V., "Remarques sur la place d'Hippocrate dans la pharmacologie de Galien", in A. DEBRU (ed.), *Galen on pharmacology: philosophy, history and medicine*, pp. 213-234, Leiden.

JOUTSIVUO, T., "Vesalius and *De humani corporis fabrica*: Galen's errors and the change of anatomy in the sixteenth century", *Hippokrates* 14, pp. 98-112.

KEYSER, P. T., "Science and magic in Galen's recipes: (sympathy and efficacy)", in A. DEBRU (ed.), *Galen on pharmacology: philosophy, history and medicine*, pp. 175-198, Leiden.

MAJUMDAR, S.K., "Galen's use of Aristotle", *Bull Indian Inst Hist Med Hyderabad.* 27.1, pp. 33-38.

MARASCO, G., "Medici alla corte dei Cesari: funzioni e metodi terapeutici", *Medizinhistorisches Journal* 32, pp. 279-297.

MARGANNE, M.-H., "Les médicaments estampillés dans le corpus galénique", in A. DEBRU (ed.), *Galen on pharmacology: philosophy, history and medicine*, pp. 153-174, Leiden.

MASSRY, S.G. et al., "Influence of Judaism and Jewish physicians on Greek and Byzantine medicine and their contribution to nephrology", *Am J Nephrol.* 17.3-4, pp. 233-240.

McVAUGH, M., "Armengaud Blaise as a translator of Galen", in E. DUDLEY SYLLA and M. McVAUGH (eds.), *Texts and contexts in ancient and medieval Science*, pp. 115-133, Leiden.

NUTTON, V., "Galen on theriac: problems of authenticity", in A. DEBRU (ed.), *Galen on pharmacology: philosophy, history and medicine*, pp. 133-151, Leiden.

REINECKE, M., *Galen und Vesal: ein Vergleich der anatomisch-physiologischen Schriften*. Münster.

ROCCA, J., "Galen and the ventricular system", *J Hist Neurosci.* 6.3, pp. 227-239.

SALAZAR, C. F., "Fragments of lost Hippocratic writings in Galen's glossary", *CQ* 47.2, pp. 543-547.

SINGER, P. N., "Levels of explanation in Galen", *CQ* 47.2, pp. 525-542.

STEIN, M., "La thériaque chez Galien: sa préparation et son usage thérapeutique", in A. DEBRU (ed.), *Galen on pharmacology: philosophy, history and medicine*, pp. 199-209, Leiden.

TOUWAIDE, A., "La thérapeutique médicamenteuse de Dioscoride à Galien: du pharmaco-centrisme au médico-centrisme", in A. DEBRU (ed.), *Galen on pharmacology: philosophy, history and medicine*, pp. 255-282, Leiden.

VON STADEN, H., "Inefficacy, error, and failure: Galen on δόκιμα φάρμακα ἄπρακτα", in A. DEBRU (ed.), *Galen on pharmacology: philosophy, history and medicine*, pp. 59-83, Leiden.

— "Galen and the «Second Sophistic»", in R. SORABJI (ed.), *Aristotle and after*, pp. 33-54, London.

1996

BAUER, A.W., "Between symbol and symptom: pain and its meanings in classical antiquity", *Schmerz.* 10.4, pp. 169-175.

DE LAUDE, S., "Picasso, Galeno, un emblema dell'Alciato", *Annali della Scuola normale superiore di Pisa, Classe di lettere e filosofia* 4.1, pp. 469-474.

DEBRU , A., *Le corps respirant: la pensée physiologique chez Galien*. Leiden.

DURLING, R. J., "ἄταρ οὖν καί in Galen and his predecessors", *Glotta* 73, p. 76.

EPSTEIN, L.C., "Medice, *cure te ipsum*: lessons from Galen", *Med Health R I.* 79.12, pp. 426-427.

FORTUNA, S., "Aspetti della tradizione del *De locis affectis* di Galeno nel rinascimento", in S. GASTALDI and M. VEGETTI (eds.), *Studi di storia della medicina antica e medievale in onore di Paola Manuli*, pp. 101-111, Florence.

GARCÍA NOVO, E., "Composition et style du traité de Galien *De inaequali intemperie*: avantages et désavantages pour la transmission du texte", in A. GARZYA and J. JOUANNA (eds.), *Histoire et ecdotique des textes médicaux grecs*, pp. 141-153, Naples.

GARCÍA SOLA, Mª.C., "Bibliografía de Galeno", *Tempus* 14, pp. 5-46.

GAROFALO, I., "Una nuova testimonianza su Ione di Chio", *FAM* 10, pp. 97-99.

GARZYA, A. and JOUANNA, J. (eds.), *Histoire et ecdotique des textes médicaux grecs*. Naples.

GASTALDI, S. and VEGETTI, M. (eds.), *Studi di storia della medicina antica e medievale in onore di Paola Manuli*. Florence.

IERACI BIO, A.Mª., "Due citazioni di Ippocrate e Galeno nell'epistola 101 K.-D. di Michele Psello", *FAM* 11, pp. 101-106.

IRIGOIN, J., "Autour des sources manuscrites de l'édition princeps de Galien", in A. GARZYA and J. JOUANNA (eds.), *Histoire et ecdotique des textes médicaux grecs*, pp. 207-216, Naples.

JACQUES, J.-M., "À propos de l'édition des fragments des médecins grecs transmis par les œuvres pharmacologiques de Galien", in A. GARZYA and J. JOUANNA (eds.), *Histoire et ecdotique des textes médicaux grecs*, pp. 236-251, Naples.

LAÍN ENTRALGO, P., "From Galen to magnetic resonance: history of medicine in Latin America", *J Med Philos.* 21.6, pp. 571 591.

LARRAIN, C.J., "Kommentar zu Galen «*De motibus dubiis*» in der mittelalterlichen Lateinischen Übersetzung des Niccolò da Reggio", *Traditio* 51, pp. 1-41.

LLOYD, G. E. R., "Theories and practices of demonstration in Galen", in M. FREDE and G. STRIKER (eds.), *Rationality in Greek thought*, pp. 255-277, Oxford.

LONGO, O., "Hot heads and cold brains: Aristotle, Galen and the «radiator theory»", *Physis* 33.1-3, pp. 259-266.

LÓPEZ FÉREZ, J.A., "Observaciones filológicas útiles para la crítica textual y la ecdótica de Galeno", in A. GARZYA and J. JOUANNA (eds.), *Histoire et ecdotique des textes médicaux grecs*, pp. 273-288, Naples.

MAGDELAINE, C., "Le commentaire de Damascius aux *Aphorismes* d'Hippocrate", in A. GARZYA and J. JOUANNA (eds.), *Histoire et ecdotique des textes médicaux grecs*, pp. 289-306, Naples.

MANETTI, D. and ROSELLI, A., "Note per una nuova edizione dei commenti di Galeno ai trattati chirurgici di Ippocrate", in S. GASTALDI and M. VEGETTI (eds.), *Studi di storia della medicina antica e medievale in onore di Paola Manuli*, pp. 77-87, Florence.

MAVROUDIS, A. D., "Galen, Περι τῶν ἰδίων βιβλίων 2", *Hellenica* 46.1, pp. 142-144.

— "The classification of the works of Galen in his treatise *On his own works*: (observations on Περι τῶν ἰδίων βιβλίων)", *Hellenica* 46.2, pp. 271-281.

MONTERO, S., "Medicina y superstición en el Africa romana: la hechicera «Favilla»", in M. KHANOUSSI; P. RUGGERI and C. VISMARA (eds.), *L'Africa romana*, pp. 403-408, Ozieri.

MUSITELLI, S., "Pagine di odontoiatria e di odontologia nel mondo antico", *MedSec* 8.2, pp. 207-235.

PIPERNO, D., "Celsus and Galen: a roman vision of respiration", *Rev Prat.* 46.11, pp. 1323-1327.

PRIORESCHI, P., "*Galenicae Quaestiones Disputatae Duae*: *rete mirabile* and pulmonary circulation", *Vesalius* 2.2, pp. 67-78.

ROOS, D.B., "Historical perspectives and anatomic considerations. Thoracic outlet syndrome", *Semin Thorac Cardiovasc Surg.* 8.2, pp. 183-189.

ROSELLI, A., "Note sulla tradizione dei commenti di Galeno ai trattati chirurgici di Ippocrate: l'apporto degli scoli ad Oribasio", in A. GARZYA and J. JOUANNA (eds.), *Histoire et ecdotique des textes médicaux grecs*, pp. 375-388, Naples.

SALMÓN, F., "Sources for a Galenic visual theory in late thirteenth century", *Sudhoffs Arch.* 80.2, pp. 167-183.

SENZASONO, L., "Limiti del platonismo in Galeno", *Metalogicon* 9.1, pp. 9-90.

STIEFEL, F. and GUEX, P., "Cancer and the mind -do we still believe Galen?", *Eur J Cancer.* 32.12, p. 2041.

SULLIVAN, R., "Thales to Galen: a brief journey through rational medical philosophy in ancient Greece. Part I: pre-Hippocratic medicine", *Proc R Coll Physicians Edinb.* 26.1, pp. 135-142.

— "Thales to Galen: a brief journey through rational medical philosophy in ancient Greece. Part II: Hippocratic medicine", *Proc R Coll Physicians Edinb.* 26.2, pp. 309-315.

— "Thales to Galen: a brief journey through rational medical philosophy in ancient Greece. Part III: Galenic medicine", *Proc R Coll Physicians Edinb.* 26.3, pp. 487-499.

TIELEMAN, T., *Galen and Chrysippus on the soul: argument and refutation in the De Placitis, Books II-III.* Leiden.

— "The hunt for Galen's shadow: Alexander of Aphrodisias, «*De anima*» 94.7-100.17 Bruns reconsidered", in K. ALGR; P.W. VAN DER HORST and D. RUNIA (eds.), *Polyhistor: studies in the history and historiography of ancient philosophy*, pp. 265-283, Leiden.

VARELLA, E.A., "Experimental techniques and laboratory apparatus in ancient Greece: drug and perfume preparation", *MedSec.* 8.2, pp. 191-206.

1995

AWAD, I.A., "Galen's anecdote of the fallen sophist: on the certainty of science through anatomy", *J Neurosurg.* 83.5, pp. 929-932.

BANNERT, H., "Galen von Pergamon, Wie man Simulanten überführt", *WHB* 37, pp. 40-49.

BEDNARCZYK, A., *Galen: glowne kategorie systemu filozoficzno-lekarskiego.* Warsaw.

BÉGUIN, D., "The problem of knowledge in Galen's *De optima doctrina*", *REG* 108, pp. 107-27.

BOUDON-MILLOT, V., "L'apport des sources arabes à la biographie de Galien", in Ph. BRUNET and M.-P. NÖEL (eds.), *Vies anciennes d' auteurs grecs: mythe et biographie*, pp. 61-79, Tours.

DEBRU, A., "Les démonstrations médicales à Rome au temps de Galien", in P.J. EIJK; H.F.J. HORTSMANSHOFF and P.H. SCRIJVERS (eds.), *Ancient Medicine in its social cultural context*, pp. 69-82, Amsterdam-Atlanta.

DERENNE, J. et al. "History of diaphragm physiology: the achievements of Galen", *Eur Respir J.* 8.1, pp. 154-160.

DURLING, R., "Method in Galen", *Dynamis* 15, pp. 41-46.

EIJK, P.J.; HORSTMANSHOFF, H.F.J. and SCHRIJVERS, P.H. (eds.), *Ancient medicine in its socio-cultural context* (2 vols.). Amsterdam-Atlanta.

GARCÍA BALLESTER, L., "Elementos para la construcción de las historias clínicas en Galeno", *Dynamis* 15, pp. 47-65.

GARCÍA BALLESTER, L.; SALMÓN, F. and SÁNCHEZ SALOR, E., "Tradición manuscrita y autoría: sobre la posible autenticidad del comentario de Arnau de Vilanova al *De morbo et accidenti* de Galeno", *Arxiu de textos catalans antics* 14, pp. 31-74.

GAROFALO, I., "La traduzione araba del *De locis affectis* di Galeno", *SCO* 45, pp. 13-63.

GUARDASOLE, A., "Per la posizione di Eraclide di Taranto nella storia del pensiero medico", *Koinonia* 19, pp. 63-69.

GYSEL, C., "Corneille De Baersdorp (1486-1565), chief physician of Charles V and commentator of Galen", *Acta Belg Hist Med.* 8, pp. 2-8.

HANKINSON, R.J., "Pollution and infection: an hypothesis still-born", *Apeiron* 28.1, pp. 25-65.

— "The growth of medical empiricism", in D. BATES (ed.), *Knowledge and the scholarly medical traditions*, pp. 60-83, Cambridge.

HORSTMANSHOFF, H.F.J., "Galen and his patients", in P.J. EIJK; H.F.J. HORSTMANSHOFF and P.H. SCHRIJVERS (eds.), *Ancient Medicine in its socio-cultural context*, pp. 83-99, Amsterdam-Atlanta.

IERODIAKONOU, K., "Alexander of Aphrodisias on medicine as a stochastic art", *CM* 28, pp. 473-485.

KURIYAMA, S., "Interpreting the history of bloodletting", *J Hist Med Allied Sci.* 50.1, pp. 11-46.

LONGO, O., "Il nome del cervello: Galeno contro Aristotele", *AAPat* 107, pp. 131-134.

MANETTI, D., "Commentarium in *Galeni De sectis*: PBerol inv. 11739; *Commentarium in Hippocratis De alimento*: *PFlor* 115", in V.V.A.A., *Corpus dei Papiri Filosofici Greci e Latini, Parte III*, pp. 19-38, 39-51, Florence.

MARASCO, G., "L' introduction de la médicine grecque à Rome: une dissension politique et idéologique", in P.J. EIJK; H.F.J. HORSTMANSHOFF and P.H. SCHRIJVERS (eds.), *Ancient medicine and its socio-cultural context*, pp. 35-48, Amsterdam-Atlanta.

MORENO RODRÍGUEZ, R.Mª., "Medicina y método científico en el mundo romano: introducción", *Dynamis* 15, pp. 19-24.

— "La ideación científica del ser mujer: uso metafórico en la doctrina galénica", *Dynamis* 15, pp. 103-145.

NUTTON, V., "Galen «*Ad multos annos*»", *Dynamis* 15, pp. 25-39.

— "Galen and the traveller's fare", in J. WILKINS; D. HARVEY and M. DOBSON (eds.), *Food in antiquity*, pp. 359-370, Exeter.

— "A new fragment of Posidonius?", *CQ* 45.1, pp. 261-263.

NUTTON, V. et al. (eds.), *The Western medical tradition, 800 B.C. to AD 1800*. Cambridge.

ROSA, P., "Per un'edizione critica del *De motu musculorum* di Galeno", *Eikasmos* 6, pp. 221-239.

SAURET, V., "On how Galen corrected a diagnosis of pleurisy", *J.Arch Bronconeumol.* 31.5, pp. 233-234.

SCHRIER, O. J., "Hunayn ibn Ishaq on tragedy and comedy: a new fragment of Galen", *Mnemosyne* 48.3, pp. 344-348.

SLUITER, I., "The poetics of medicine", in J. ABBENES; S. SLINGS and I. SLUITER (eds.), *Greek literary theory after Aristotle*, pp. 193-213, Amsterdam.

— "The embarrassment of imperfection: Galen's assessment of Hippocrates' linguistic merits", *CM* 28, pp. 519-535.

THIVEL, A., "Theorie und Empirie in der römischen Medizin und bei Galen", in B. KÜHNERT; V. RIEDEL and R. GORDESIANI (eds.), *Prinzipat und Kultur im 1. und 2. Jahrhundert*, pp. 90-99, Amsterdam.

TIELEMAN, T., "Dialectic and science: Galen, Herophilus and Aristotle on phenomena", *CM* 28, pp. 487-495.

— "Galen on the seat of the mind: medical experiment and philosophical tradition", *Gewina* 18.3, pp. 24-36.

TOUWAIDE, A., "L'integration de la pharmacologie grecque dans le monde arabe: une vue d'ensemble", *MedSec* 7.1, pp. 159-189.

— "A conference on the pharmacology of Galen", *Rev Hist Pharm* 42 (nº 307), pp. 377-380.

VEGETTI, M., "Galeno e la rifondazione della medicina", *Dynamis* 15, pp. 67-101.

VIGLIANI, R., "Galen's oncology", *Pathologica* 87.5, pp. 577-590.

VON STADEN, H., "Science as text, science as history: Galen on metaphor", *CM* 28, pp. 499-518.

— "Anatomy as rhetoric: Galen on dissection and persuasion", *J Hist Med Allied Sci.* 50.1, pp. 47-66.

ZONTA, M., *Un interprete ebreo della filosofia di Galeno: gli scritti filosofici di Galeno nell'opera di Shem Tob ibn Falaquera.* Torino

1994

ANDRÁS, L., "Galen: the good physician is also a philosopher", *Orv Hetil* 135 (nº 44), pp. 2437-2438.

BOUDON-MILLOT, V., "Loisir et création littéraire chez Galien", *Bulletin de l'Association Guillaume Budé* 2, pp. 154-168.

— "Les oeuvres de Galien pour les débutants (*De sectis, De pulsibus ad tirones, De ossibus ad tirones, Ad Glauconem de método medendi* et *Ars medica*): médicine et pédagogie au IIe siècle après J.-C.", in W. HASSE (ed.), *ANRW* 37.2, pp. 1421-1467, Berlin.

— *L'apport des sources arabes à la biographie de Galien.* Tours.

BRUNT, P., "The bubble of the Second Sophistic", *BICS* 39, pp. 25-52.

DEBRU, A., "L'expérimentation chez Galien", in W. HAASE (ed.), *ANRW* II, 37.2, pp.1718-1756, Berlin.

FINKIELMAN, S., "Between Hippocrates and Galen", *Medicina* 54.4, pp. 371-3.

FREEMON F.R., "Galen's ideas on neurological function", *J Hist Neurosci.* 3.4, pp. 263-71.

FRIEDRICH, C., "Von der Galenik zur modernen pharmazeutischen Technologie Historische Entwicklung und Ausblick", *Pharmazie* 49.5, 307-312.

GARCÍA BALLESTER, L., *Tradición e innovación en el helenismo: su uso en la medicina por Galeno.* Malaga.

— "Galen as a clinician: his methods in diagnostics", in W. HAASE (ed.), *ANRW* II, 37.2, pp. 1636-1671, Berlin.

GRMEK, M.D. and GOUREVITCH, D., "Aux sources de la doctrine médicale de Galien: l'enseignement de Marinus, Quintus et Numisianus", in W. HAASE (ed.), *ANRW* II, 37.2, pp. 1491-1528, Berlin.

HALFWASSEN, J., "Bemerkungen zum Ursprung der Lehre vom Seelenwagen", *JRTR* 2, pp. 114-128.

HANKINSON, R.J., "Galen and the logic of relations", in L.P. SCHRENK (ed.), *Aristotle in Late Antiquity*, pp. 57-75, Washington.

— "Usage and abusage: Galen on language", in S. EVERSON (ed.), *Language*, pp. 166-187, Cambridge.

— "Galen's theory of causation", in W. HAASE (ed.), *ANRW* II, 37.2, pp. 1757-1774, Berlin.

— "Galen's concept of scientific progress", in W. HAASE (ed.), *ANRW* II, 37.2, pp. 1775-1789, Berlin.

— "Galen's Anatomical procedures: a second-century debate in medical epistemology", in W. HAASE (ed.), *ANRW* II, 37.2, pp. 1834-1855, Berlin.

HIATT, J.R. and HIATT, N., "Galen -a father of medicine", *J Am Coll Surg*. 178.4, pp. 410-416.

KARENBERG A., "Reconstructing a doctrine: Galen on apoplexy", *J Hist Neurosci*. 3.2, pp. 85-101.

KOLLESCH, J., "Die Sprache von Arzten nichtgriechischer Herkunft im Urteil Galens", *Philologus* 138.2, pp. 260-263.

LARRAIN, C.J., "Galen, «*De motibus dubiis*»: Übersetzung des Niccolò da Reggio", *Traditio* 49, pp. 171-233.

MANETTI, D. and ROSELLI, A., "Galeno commentatore di Ippocrate", in W. HAASE (ed.), *ANRW* II, 37.2, pp. 1529-1635, Berlin.

PRIORESCHI, P., "Experimentation and scientific method in the classical world: their rise and decline", *Med Hypotheses* 42.3, pp. 135-48.

QUIN, C.E., "The soul and the pneuma in the function of the nervous system after Galen", *J R Soc Med*. 87.7, pp. 393-395.

SLUITER, I., "Two problems in ancient medical commentaries", *CQ* 44.1, pp. 270 275.

TOUWAIDE, A., "Galien et la toxicologie", in W. HAASE (ed.), *ANRW* II, 37.2, pp. 1887-1986, Berlin.

TZORTZATOU-STATHOPOULOU, F.,"History of pediatric hematology and oncology in Greece", *Pediatr Hematol Oncol*. 11.1, pp. 13-25.

VEGETTI, M., "L'imagine del medico e lo statuto epistemologico della medicina in Galeno", in W. HAASE (ed.), *ANRW* II, 37.2, pp. 1672-1717, Berlin.

1993

BARNES, J., "«A third sort of syllogism»: Galen and the logic of relations", in R.W. SHARPLES (ed.), *Modern thinkers and ancient thinkers*, pp. 172-194, London.

— "Galen and the utility of logic", in J. KOLLESCH and D. NICKEL (eds.), *Galen und das hellenistische Erbe*, pp. 33-52, Stuttgart.

BERKA, K., "Galen: Arzt und Logiker", *GLP* 14, pp. 15-20.

BLUM, J.H., "Galen and the Judeo-Christian tradition: reflections on Galen's attitude toward critical examination", *Korot* 10, pp. 115-134.

BOMPAIRE, J., "Quatre styles d'autobiographie au IIe siècle après J.-C.: Aelius Aristide, Lucien, Marc Aurèle, Galien", in M.F. BASLEZ; Ph. HOFFMANN and L. PERNOT (eds.), *L'invention de l'autobiographie d'Hésiode à Saint Augustin*, pp. 199-209, Paris.

BOUDON-MILLOT, V., "Medicine and teaching in Galen's *Ars medica*", *REG* 106, pp. 120-141.

BYL, S., "From Hippocrates to Galen", *Acta Belg Hist Med.* 6.3, pp. 141-149.

CORBAN, A., "Galen, the solitary master", *Bull Soc Liban Hist Med.* 1, pp. 1-7.

DURLING, R.J., *A Dictionary of medical terms in Galen*. Leiden.

EIJK, P.J., "A textual note on Galen, on the powers of foodstuffs I 1.3 (P. 202.17 Helmreich)", *CQ* 43.2, pp. 506-508.

FORTUNA, S., "Galen's "*De constitutione artis medicinae*" in the Renaissance", *CQ* 43.1, pp. 302-319.

GARCÍA BALLESTER, L., "On the origin of the «six non-natural things» in Galen", in J. KOLLESCH and D. NICKEL (eds.), *Galen und das hellenistische Erbe*, pp. 105-115, Stuttgart.

GIL SOTRES, P., "Le regole della salute", in M.D. GRMEK (ed.), *Storia del pensiero medico occidentale*, pp. 399-438, Rome.

GOUREVITCH, D., "Le vie della conoscenza: la medicina nel mondo romano", in M.D. GRMEK (ed.), *Storia del pensiero medico occidentale*, pp. 121-165, Rome.

GRENSEMANN, H., "Peliás, Columba livia, die Felsentaube, als Krankheitsname", *ZWG* 77.1, pp. 114-116.

GRMEK, M.D., "Il concetto di malattia", in M.D. GRMEK (ed.), *Storia del pensiero medico occidentale*, pp. 323-347, Rome.

HANKINSON, R.J., "Actions and passions: affection, emotion, and moral self-management in Galen's philosophical psychology", in J. BRUNSCHWIG and M. NUSSBAUM (eds.), *Passions and perceptions: studies in Hellenistic philosophy of mind*, pp. 184-222, Cambridge.

JACQUART, D., "La scolastica medica", in M.D. GRMEK (ed.), *Storia del pensiero medico occidentale*, pp. 261-321, Rome.

JOUANNA, J., "La nascita dell' arte medica occidentale", in M.D. GRMEK (ed.), *Storia del pensiero medico occidentale*, pp. 3-72, Rome.

JOUANNA, J. and BOUDON-MILLOT, V., "Defense and illustration of Classical Humanism: a presentation on a project towards an edition of Galen in the collections of the University of Paris", *Bulletin de l'Association Guillaume Budé*, 2, pp. 101-135.

KOLLESCH, J., "Eine hippokratische Krankheitseinteilung in den pseudogatenischen *Definitiones medicae*", in P. POTTER; G. MALONEY and J. DESAUTES (eds.), *Actes VI Colloque international Hippocratique*, pp. 255-264, Quebec.

KOLLESCH, J. and NICKEL, D. (eds.), *Galen und das hellenistische Erbe*. Stuttgart.

LARRAIN, C.J., "Ein bislang unbekanntes griechisches Fragment der Galen zugeschriebenen Schrift *Peri aporon kineseon* (*De motibus dubiis*)", *Philologus* 137.2, pp. 265-273.

LLOYD, G.E.R., "Galen on Hellenistics and Hippocrateans: contemporary battles and past authorities", in J. KOLLESCH and D. NICKEL (eds.), *Galen und das hellenistische Erbe Galen und das hellenistische Erbe*, pp. 125-143, Stuttgart.

LÓPEZ FÉREZ, J.A., "Aspectos teóricos, empíricos y léxicos del agua en Galeno", in J. KOLLESCH and D. NICKEL (eds.), *Galen und das hellenistische Erbe Galen und das hellenistische Erbe*, pp. 173-191, Stuttgart.

MANSFELD, J., "The idea of the will in Chrysippus, Posidonius, and Galen", in J.J. CLEARY (ed.), *Proceedings of the Boston Area Colloquium in Ancient Philosophy: VII*, pp. 107-145, 153-157, Leiden.

MANULI, P., "Galen and Stoicism", in J. KOLLESCH and D. NICKEL (eds.), *Galen und das hellenistische Erbe Galen und das hellenistische Erbe*, pp. 53 61, Stuttgart.

MARÓTH, M., "Galen als Seelenheiler", in J. KOLLESCH and D. NICKEL (eds.), *Galen und das hellenistische Erbe Galen und das hellenistische Erbe*, pp. 145-155, Stuttgart.

MEZZOGIORNO, V.; MEZZOGIORNO, A., and PASSIATORE C., "A contribution to the history of renal structure knowledge (from Galen to Malpighi)", *Ann Anat*. 175.5, pp. 395-401.

NICKEL, D., "Stoa und Stoiker in Galens Schrift *De foetuum formatione*", in J. KOLLESCH and D. NICKEL (eds.), *Galen und das hellenistische Erbe Galen und das hellenistische Erbe*, pp. 79-86, Stuttgart.

NUTTON, V., "Galen and Egypt", in J. KOLLESCH and D. NICKEL (eds.), *Galen und das hellenistische Erbe Galen und das hellenistische Erbe*, pp. 11-31, Stuttgart.

ORMOS, I., "Bemerkungen zur editorischen Bearbeitung der Galenschrift Über die Sektion toter Lebewesen", in J. KOLLESCH and D. NICKEL (eds.), *Galen und das hellenistische Erbe Galen und das hellenistische Erbe*, pp. 165-172, Stuttgart.

PIGEAUD, J., "Les problèmes de la création chez Galien", in J. KOLLESCH and D. NICKEL (eds.), *Galen und das hellenistische Erbe Galen und das hellenistische Erbe*, pp. 87-103, Stuttgart.

— "Galen on the topic of creation", *Sudhoffs Arch Z Wissenschaftsgesch Beih.* 32, pp. 87-103.

POTTER, P., "Apollonius and Galen on «Joints»", in J. KOLLESCH and D. NICKEL (eds.), *Galen und das hellenistische Erbe Galen und das hellenistische Erbe*, pp. 117-123, Stuttgart.

RICHARDSON, W. F., "First find your part, then name it", *Prudentia* 25.2, pp. 29-46.

RIDDLE, J.M., "High medicine and low medicine in the Roman empire", in W. HAASE (ed.), *ANRW* II, 37.1, pp. 102-120, Berlin.

ROSNER, F., "Headache in the writings of Moses Maimonides and other Hebrew sages", *Headache* 33.6, pp. 315-319.

SALMÓN, F. and SÁNCHEZ SALOR, E., "On the use of authority in medieval medicine: Aristotle, Galen and flying flies", *Dynamis* 13, pp. 347-371.

SCARBOROUGH, J., "Roman medicine to Galen", in W. HAASE (ed.), *ANRW* II, 37.1, pp. 3-48, Berlin.

STROHMAIER, G., "Hellenistische Wissenschaft im neugefundenen Galenkommentar zur hippokratischen Schrift Über die Umwelt", in J. KOLLESCH and D. NICKEL (eds.), *Galen und das hellenistische Erbe Galen und das hellenistische Erbe*, pp. 157-164, Stuttgart.

—"La ricezione e la tradizione: la medicina nel mondo bizantino e arabo", in M.D. GRMEK (ed.), *Storia del pensiero medico occidentale*, pp. 167-215, Rome.

VARDANJAN, S.A., "Galen und die mittelalterliche armenische Medizin", in J. KOLLESCH and D. NICKEL (eds.), *Galen und das hellenistische Erbe Galen und das hellenistische Erbe*, pp. 193-203, Stuttgart.

VEGETTI, M., "I nervi dell'anima", in J. KOLLESCH and D. NICKEL (eds.), *Galen und das hellenistische Erbe Galen und das hellenistische Erbe*, pp. 63-77, Stuttgart.

1992

BARIGAZZI, A., "Ludovico Bellisario ovvero dell'uso delle versioni latine in una edizione di Galeno", in A. GARZYA (ed.), *Tradizione e ecdotica dei testi medici tardoantichi e bizantini,* pp. 29-39, Naples.

— "Un manifesto di Galeno ai medici", *Prometheus* 18, pp. 127-138.

BERTINI MALGARINI, A., "Costituzione del corpo nel *De optima corporis nostri constitutione* e nel *De bono habitu di Galeno*", in A. GARZYA (ed.), *Tradizione e ecdotica dei testi medici tardoantichi e bizantini,* pp. 41-50, Naples.

BOERI, M.D., "La transmisión del concepto estoico de causa sinéctica", *Méthexis* 5, pp. 99-121

CAPONE CIOLLARO M. and GALLI CALDERIN, I.G., "Problemi relativi alle fonti di Aezio Amideno nei libri IX-XVI: Galeno e Oribasio", in A. GARZYA (ed.), *Tradizione e ecdotica dei testi medici tardoantichi e bizantini,* pp. 51-72, Naples.

CHERUBIN, P., *A la rencontre de Galien médecin et philosophe*. Limoges.

DE LACY, Ph., "A Galenic argument", *AJPh* 113.2, pp. 275-276.

DEBRU, A., *La pensée physiologique: doctrines et langages de la respiration chez Galien à l'époque grecoromain*. Lille.

— "La suffocation hystérique chez Galien et Aétius: réécriture et emprunt du «je»", in A. GARZYA (ed.), *Tradizione e ecdotica dei testi medici tardoantichi e bizantini,* pp. 79-89, Naples.

DEMONT, P.L., "Note sur Hippocratte, *Epidémies* III, 15-16", *RHT*, pp. 253-257.

DONINI, P., "Galeno e la filosofia", W. HASSE (ed.), *ANRW* II, 36.5, pp. 3484-3504, Berlin.

DUMONT, M., "La gynécologie et l'obstetrique chez les Romains", *Rev.Fr.Gynecol.Obstet.* 87.10, pp. 493-496, 499-505.

DURAND, Ph., "Sur la construction du livre II du Περὶ ἀντιδότων de Galien", *REA* 93, pp. 99-108.

DURLING, R.J., "The language of Galenic pharmacy", *Glotta* 70, 62-70.

FARIA, M., "The forging of the Renaissance physician: a philosophic and historic perspective. Part I: The influence of Hippocrates, Galen, and Islamic physicians", *J Med Assoc Ga.* 81.3, pp. 119-123.

— "The forging of the Renaissance physician: a philosophic and historic perspective. Part II: The philosophic basis for pre-Renaissance medical knowledge", *J.Med.Assoc.Ga.* 81.3, pp. 124-126.

GAROFALO, I., "Galeno e l'anatomia di Ippocrate", in J.A. LÓPEZ FÉREZ (ed.), *Tratados hipocráticos. Estudios acerca de su contenido, forma e influencia*, pp. 609-622, Madrid.

GARZYA, A. (ed.), *Tradizione e ecdotica dei testi medici tardoantichi e bizantini.* Naples.

GRONEWALD, M., “Galen, *De antidotis* I in P. Lit. London 169”, *ZPE* 93, pp. 24-25.

HANKINSON, R.J., “Galen’s philosophical eclecticism”, W. HASSE (ed.), *ANRW* II, 36.5, pp. 3505-3522, Berlin.

HÜLSER, K., “Galen und die Logik”, W. HASSE (ed.), *ANRW* II, 36.5, pp. 3523-3554, Berlin.

IRIGOIN, J., “Traductions arabes de traités médicaux grecs et leurs différents types de sources”, in A. GARZYA (ed.), *Tradizione e ecdotica dei testi medici tardoantichi e bizantini,* pp. 147-155, Naples.

ISLER, H., “The Galenic tradition and migraine”, *J Hist Neurosci.* 1.3, pp. 227-233.

JOUANNA, J., “Les médecins grecs dans la collection Budé”, in A. GARZYA (ed.), *Tradizione e ecdotica dei testi medici tardoantichi e bizantini,* pp. 345-347, Naples.

KING, J.B., “Focal points in orthopaedics”, *Br.Med.Bull.* 48.3, pp. 651-667.

LARRAIN, C.J., *Galens Kommentar zu Platons Timaios.* Stuttgart.

LÓPEZ FÉREZ, J.A. (ed.), *Tratados hipocráticos. Estudios acerca de su contenido, forma e influencia.* Madrid.

— “Galeno, lector y crítico de manuscritos”, in A. GARZYA (ed.), *Tradizione e ecdotica dei testi medici tardoantichi e bizantini,* pp. 197-209, Naples.

MANETTI, D., “P.Berol. 11739A e i commenti tardo-antichi a Galeno”, in A. GARZYA (ed.), *Tradizione e ecdotica dei testi medici tardoantichi e bizantini,* pp. 211-235, Naples.

MANETTI, D. and ROSELLI, A., “Problemi di edizione della sezione anatomica di *Epidemie* II”, in J.A. LÓPEZ FÉREZ (ed.), *Tratados hipocráticos. Estudios acerca de su contenido, forma e influencia*, pp. 623-634, Madrid.

NUTTON, V. “The Galenic Codices of Theodore Goulston”, *RHT* 22, pp. 259-278.

VON STADEN, H., “The discovery of the body: human dissection and its cultural contexts in ancient Greece”, *Yale J Biol Med.* 65.3, pp. 223-241.

WOLSKA-CONUS, W., “Les commentaires de Stéphanos d’Athènes au *Prognostikon* et aux *Aphorismes* d’Hippocrate: de Galien à la practique scolaire alexandrine”, *REbyz* 50, pp. 5-86.

1991

BARNES, J., “Galen on logic and therapy”, in F. KUDLIEN and R.J. DURLING (eds.), *Galen's method of healing*, pp. 50-102, Leiden.

BYL, S. and BARRIGANT, A., “L'enfant chez Galien”, in J.A. LÓPEZ FÉREZ (ed.), *Galeno: obra, pensamiento e influencia*, pp. 107-117, Madrid.

BYLEBYL, J.J., “Teaching *Methodus medendi* in the Renaissance”, in F. KUDLIEN and R.J. DURLING (eds.), *Galen's method of healing*, pp. 157-189, Leiden.

CASSELS, I., “A brief note on Arabic equivalents to Galen's *Endeixis*”, *Stud Anc Med* 1, pp. 114-116.

DEBRU, A., “Expérience, plausibilité et certitude chez Galien”, in J.A. LÓPEZ FÉREZ (ed.), *Galeno: obra, pensamiento e influencia*, pp. 31-40, Madrid.

DILG, P., “Johann Agricola Ammonius' Kommentar zu Galens *Methodus medendi*”, in F. KUDLIEN and R.J. DURLING (eds.), *Galen's Method of healing*, pp. 190-198, Leiden.

FORTUNA, S., “La tradizione del *De constitutione artis medicae* di Galeno”, *BollClass* 11, pp. 48-77.

GAROFALO, I., “L'anatomia umana di Galeno”, *Rivista trismestrale di analisi e critica-Nuova civilta delle macchine* 3-4, pp. 101-111.

— “The six classes of animals in Galen”, in J.A. LÓPEZ FÉREZ (ed.), *Galeno: Obra, Pensamiento e influencia*, pp. 73-87, Madrid.

GETZ, F.M., “The method of healing in Middle English”, F. KUDLIEN and R.J. DURLING (eds.), *Galen's Method of healing*, pp. 147-156, Leiden.

GOUREVITCH, D., “L'alimentation végétal de famine dans l'Empire romain. Un témoignage de Galien”, *Acta Facultatis Medicae Fluminensis* 16, pp. 59-63.

HANKINSON, R.J., “Galen's anatomy of the soul”, *Phronesis* 36, pp. 197-233.

— “Galen on the foundation of science”, in J.A. LÓPEZ FÉREZ, J.A. (ed.), *Galeno: Obra, Pensamiento e influencia*, pp. 15-29, Madrid.

IELO, M., “Nicola Deoprepio: un greco traduttore di Ippocrate e Galeno presso la corte di Roberto d'Angiò”, *Parnasso* 33, pp. 353-356.

IERACI BIO, A.M., “Sulla concezione del medico pepaideuménos in Galeno e nel tardoantico”, in J.A. LÓPEZ FÉREZ (ed.), *Galeno: Obra, Pensamiento e influencia*, pp. 133-152, Madrid.

JOUANNA, J., “Remarques sur la tradition arabe du commentaire de Galien aux traités hippocratiques des Airs, eaux, lieux et du Serment”, in J.A. LÓPEZ FÉREZ (ed.), *Galeno: Obra, Pensamiento e influencia*, pp. 235-251, Madrid.

KIBRE, P., "A list of Latin manuscripts containing medieval versions of the *Methodus medendi*", in F. KUDLIEN and R.J. DURLING (eds.), *Galen's Method of healing*, pp. 117-122, Leiden.

KUDLIEN F., "*Endeixis* as a scientific term. Galen's usage of the word (in medicine and logic)", in F. KUDLIEN and R.J. DURLING (eds.), *Galen's Method of healing*, pp. 103-111, Leiden.

KUDLIEN F. and DURLING, R.J. (eds.), *Galen's method of healing*. Leiden.

LAÍN ENTRALGO, P., "Actualidad de Galeno. Nota sobre las *sex res non naturales*", in LÓPEZ FÉREZ, J.A. (ed.), *Galeno: Obra, Pensamiento e influencia*, pp. 11-14, Madrid.

LARA NAVA, D., "Aspectos lexicográficos del glosario de Galeno a Hipócrates", in J.A. LÓPEZ FÉREZ (ed.), *Galeno: Obra, Pensamiento e influencia*, pp. 119-131, Madrid.

LARRAIN, C.J., "Ein unbekanntes Exzerpt aus Galens *Timaiokommentar*", *ZPE* 85, pp. 9-30.

LÓPEZ EIRE, J.A., "Sobre el eclecticismo de Galeno", in J.A. LÓPEZ FÉREZ (ed.), *Galeno: Obra, Pensamiento e influencia*, pp. 57-72, Madrid.

LÓPEZ FÉREZ, J.A. (ed.), *Galeno: Obra, pensamiento e influencia*. Madrid.

— "Acerca del comentario de Galeno a los *Aforismos* hipocráticos", in J.A. LÓPEZ FÉREZ (ed.), *Galeno: Obra, Pensamiento e influencia*, pp. 161-203, Madrid.

— "Ediciones de Galeno. Bibliografía", in J.A. LÓPEZ FÉREZ (ed.), *Galeno: Obra, Pensamiento e influencia*, pp. 306-337, Madrid.

—"Le témoignage de Galien sur les méthodiques à Rome", in Ph. MURRAY and J. PIGEAUD (eds.), *Actes du 2ème colloque international sur les textes médicaux antiques*, pp. 187-201, Geneve.

MANI, N., "Die Wissenschaftliche Grundlagen der Chirurgie bei Galen", in F. KUDLIEN and R.J. DURLING (eds.), *Galen's Method of healing*, pp. 26-49, Leiden.

MANULI, P., "Galen and Stoicism", in F. KUDLIEN and R.J. DURLING (eds.), *Galen's Method of healing*, pp. 53-61, Leiden.

MESTRE, F., "Galén: l'autobiografia d'un home de ciencia", in L. FERRERES (ed.), *Mélanges V. Bejarano* II, pp. 673-677, Barcelona.

MORENO RODRÍGUEZ, R.Mª., "Una interpretación no humoralista de la estequiología galénica", in J.A. LÓPEZ FÉREZ (ed.), *Galeno: Obra, Pensamiento e influencia*, pp. 89-105, Madrid.

NUTTON, V., "Style and context in the method of healing", in F. KUDLIEN and R.J. DURLING (eds.), *Galen's Method of healing*, pp. 1-25, Leiden.

PIÑERO, F., "Galeno y las referencias de Maimónides a Epicuro en el *Morch nevuchim* (*Guía de perplejos*)", in J.A. LÓPEZ FÉREZ (ed.), *Galeno: Obra, Pensamiento e influencia*, pp. 273-279, Madrid.

SANTANA HENRÍQUEZ, G., "En torno a la composición en la prosa médica griega antigua", *Emerita* 59, pp. 123-132.

SCOTT, A., "Ps-Thessalus of Tralles and Galen's *De methodo medendi*", *ZWG* 75, pp. 10-110.

SIMMS, D.L., "Galen on Archimedes: burning mirror or burning pitch", *T&C* 32, pp. 91-96.

SINGER, P.N., "Aspects of Galen's Platonism", in J.A. LÓPEZ FÉREZ (ed.), *Galeno: Obra, Pensamiento e influencia*, pp. 41-55, Madrid.

VÁZQUEZ BUJAN, M.E., "Notas sobre la pervivencia tardolatina de Galeno", in J.A. LÓPEZ FÉREZ (ed.), *Galeno: Obra, Pensamiento e influencia*, pp. 223-233, Madrid.

VON STADEN, H., "Galen as historian: his use of sources on the Herophileans", in J.A. LÓPEZ FÉREZ (ed.), *Galeno: Obra, Pensamiento e influencia*, pp. 205-222, Madrid.

WEISSERE, U., "Zur Rezeption der *Methodus medendi* im continens des Rhazes", in F. KUDLIEN and R.J. DURLING (eds.), *Galen's Method of healing*, pp. 123-143, Leiden.

— "Hippokrates (ca. 460-ca. 375 v. Chr.), Galen (129-ca. 200 oder nach n. Chr.)", in D. ENGELHARDT and F. HARTMANN (eds.), *Klassiker der Medezin I*, pp. 11-20, Munich.

1990

GERO, S., "Galen on the Christians: a reappraisal of the Arabic evidence", *OCP* 56, pp. 371-411.

GITTER, A.H., "Eine kurze Geschichte der Horforschung I. Antike", *Laryngorhinootologie* 69, pp. 442-445.

GRINHNASCHI, M., "Il catalogo delle opere di Ippocrate e Galeno nel *Vita et moribus philosophorum*", *Medioevo* 16, pp. 355-395.

MAGNALDI, G., "Per un'edizione critica del περὶ παθῶν di Galeno", *Bollettino dei Classici* 11, pp. 5-47.

NUTTON, V., "The patien's choice: a new treatise by Galen", *CQ* 40, pp. 236-257.

1989

BÉGUIN, D., "L'édition Goulston et les prétendus manuscrits perdus de Galien", *RHT* 19, pp. 341-349.

FORTUNA, S., "*Par. Gr.* 2308 et *Par. Gr.* 2269: testimoni del *Dignotione ex insomniis* e del *De Praecognitione* di Galeno", *SCO* 39, pp. 353-354.

HANKINSON, R.J., "Galen and the best of all possible worlds", *CQ* 39, pp. 206-227.

HIATT, N. and HIATT, J.R., "Galen and the greatest medical book", *Pharos* 52, pp. 24-26.

IRIGOIN, J., "Tradition et critique des textes grecs", *ACF* 81, pp. 585-605.

JENNER, K.A., *A study of Galen's Commentary on the Prognostikon of Hippocrates*. Oxford.

LANATA, G., "L'Inmortalità artificiale. Appunti sul proemio della *Novella* 22 di Giustiniano", *Serta historica Antiqua* 2, pp. 259-263.

MALATESTA, M., "An extension of Genttzen's natural deduction", *Metalogicon* 2, pp. 1-32.

— "Classical fundamentals and a modern foundation of the probability calculus", *Metalogicon* 2, pp. 94-132.

MORO, F.; MIDENA, E. and PREMUDA, L., "The anatomy and physiology of the optic nerve: historical notes", *Metab.Pediatr.Syst. Ophthalmol* 12, pp. 7-12.

REPICI, L., "L'epiglottide nell'antichita: tra medicina e filosofia", *HPLS* 12, pp. 67-104.

SCARBOROUGH, J., "Pharmaceutical theory in Galen's commentaries on the Hippocratic *Epidemics*: some observations on Roman views of Greek drug lore", *ZWG* 27, pp. 270-282.

SCHERENE, L.P., "Byzantine evidence for Galen's *On medical experience*", *ByzZ* 82, pp. 251-257.

SMITH, W.D., "Notes on ancient medical historiography", *BHM* 63, pp. 73-109.

SORETH, M., "Die galenischen Kettenschlussfiguren als Figuren von Kettenschlüssen mit vier Termen", *AGPh* 71, pp. 175-215.

TILLES, G. and WALLACH, D., "Histoire de la nosologie en dermatologie", *Ann.Dermatol.Venereol* 116, pp. 9-26.

VON STADEN, H., *Herophilus. The Art of Medicine in Early Alexandria*. Cambridge.

WASSERSTEIN, D.J., "Greek science in Islam, Islamic scholars as succesors to the Greek", *Hermathena* 147, pp. 57-72.

WITTERN, R., "Die Wechselfieber bei Galen" *HPLS* 11, pp. 3-22.

1988

ACHTÉ, K. and KARHA, E., "Galen and psychiatry", *Hippokrates* 5, pp. 70-79.

BONNET-CADILHAC, C., "Connaissances de Galien sur l'anatomo-physiologie de l'appareil genital feminin", *HPLS* 10, pp. 267-291.

BOUDON-MILLOT, V., "Galien et le sacré", *Bulletin de l'Association Guillaume Budé* 47, pp. 327-337.

BYL, S., "La gerontologie de Galien", *HPLS* 10, pp. 73-92.

DE LACY, Ph., "The third part of the soul", in P. MANULI and M. VEGETTI (eds.), *Le opere psicologiche di Galeno. Atti del terzo colloquio galenico internazionale*, pp. 43-63, Naples.

DIEPPE, P., "Did Galen describe rheumatoid arthritis? [letter]", *Ann. Rheum. Dis* 47, pp. 84-85.

DOLS, M.W., "Galen and Islamic psychiatry", in P. MANULI and M. VEGETTI (eds.), *Le opere psicologiche di Galeno. Atti del terzo colloquio galenico internazionale*, pp. 243-280, Naples.

DONINI, P., "Tipologia degli errore e loro correzione secondo Galeno", in P. MANULI and M. VEGETTI (eds.), *Le opere psicologiche di Galeno. Atti del terzo colloquio galenico internazionale*, pp. 65-116, Naples.

DURLING, R.J., "Some particles and particle clusters in Galen", *Glotta* 66, pp. 183-189.

— "The innate heat in Galen", *MHJ* 23, p. 210.

FEUGERE, M., et al. "L'opération de la cataracte dans le monde romain et l'intrumentarium de Montbellet", *Doss. Arch.* 123, pp. 67-71.

GARCÍA BALLESTER, L., "Soul and body, disease of the soul and disease of the body in Galen's medical thought", in P. MANULI and M. VEGETTI (eds.), *Le opere psicologiche di Galeno. Atti del terzo colloquio galenico internazionale*, pp. 117-152, Naples.

GOUREVITCH, D., "Galien, médecin-décideur. Déjouer les pièges tendus par les malades", *Prospective et Santé* 46, pp. 81-88.

GUGGENHEIM, K.Y., "Galen of Pergamon on obesity", *Koroth* 9.7-8, pp. 555-556.

HANKINSON, R.J., "Galien: la médecine et la philosophie antisceptique", *RPhA* 6, pp. 229-269.

JACQUART, D., "Représentations de Galien dans la peinture médievale", *Dossiers Histoire et Archéologie* 123, pp. 22-29.

KOLLESCH, J., "Anschauungen von der archaí in der *Ars medica* und die Seelehre Galens", in P. MANULI and M. VEGETTI (eds.), *Le opere psicologiche di Galeno. Atti del terzo colloquio galenico internazionale*, pp. 215-229, Naples.

LASCARATOS, J. and MARKETOS, S., "A historical outline of Greek ophthalmology from the Hellenistic period up to the establishment of the first universities", *Doc.Ophthalmol* 68, pp. 157-169.

LLOYD, G.E.R., "Scholarship, authority and argument in Galen's *Quod animi mores*", in P. MANULI and M. VEGETTI (eds.), *Le opere psicologiche di Galeno. Atti del terzo colloquio galenico internazionale*, pp. 11-42, Naples.

LÓPEZ FÉREZ, J.A., "L'animal dans l'alimentation humaine selon Galien", in L. BODSON (ed.), *L'animal dans l'alimentation*, pp. 91-94, Paris.

MANI, N., "Physiologische Konzepte von Galen bis Haller", *Gesnerus* 45, pp. 165-190.

MANULI, P. and VEGETTI, M. (eds.), *Le opere psicologiche di Galeno. Atti del terzo colloquio galenico internazionale*. Naples.

MANULI, P., "La passione nel *De placitis Hippocratis et Platonis*", in P. MANULI and M. VEGETTI (eds.), *Le opere psicologiche di Galeno. Atti del terzo colloquio galenico internazionale*, pp. 185-214, Naples.

NUTTON, V., "Galens' *De placitis Hippocratis et Platonis* in the Renaissance", in P. MANULI and M. VEGETTI (eds.), *Le opere psicologiche di Galeno. Atti del terzo colloquio galenico internazionale*, pp. 281-309, Naples.

PIGEAUD, J., "La psychopatologie de Galien", in P. MANULI and M. VEGETTI (eds.), *Le opere psicologiche di Galeno. Atti del terzo colloquio galenico internazionale*, pp. 153-183, Naples.

POUDERON, B., "La chaîne alimentaire chez Athénagore. Cofrontation de sa théorie digestive avec la science médicale de son temps", *Orpheus* 9, pp. 219-237.

SCARBOROUGH, J., "Galen redivivus", *JHM* 43, pp. 313-321

STROHMAIER, G., "Avicennas Lehre von den "inneren Sinnen" und ihre Voraussetzungen bei Galen", in P. MANULI and M. VEGETTI (eds.), *Le opere psicologiche di Galeno. Atti del terzo colloquio galenico internazionale*, pp. 231-242, Naples.

VON STADEN, H., *Herophilus: the art of medicine in early Alexandria*. Cambridge.

1987

ACCANTINO, P., "*Ematopoiesi.* Malattia cardiaca e disturbi mentali in Galeno e in Alessandro di Afrodisia", *Hermes* 15, pp. 454-473.

ANDRÉ, J.-M., *Être médecin à Rome*. Paris.

CASSIO, A.C., "I tempi di composizione delle comedie attiche e una parafrasi di Aristofane in Galeno", *RFIC* 115, pp. 5-11.

CENTANNI, M., "Nomi del male. Phrenitis e epilepsia nel *Corpus Galenicum*", *MusPat* 5, pp. 47-49.

CHRISTIE, R.V., "Galen on Erasistratus", *Perspect.Biol.Med* 30, pp. 440-449.

DEBRU, A., "Galien commentateur d'Hippocrate: le canon hippocratique", in C. IMBERT-VALASSOPOULOS and R. TRIAU (eds.), *Hippocrate et son héritage Colloque franco-hellénique d'histoire de la médecine*, pp. 51-56, Lyon.

FORTUNA, S., "La definizione della medicina in Galeno", *PP* 42, pp. 181-196.

GELPKE, A., *Das Koncept des erkrankten Ortes in Galens De locis affectis*. Zurich.

GERICKE, D., "Hippokrates und Galenos diskutieren", *Fortschr. Med* 105, p. 64.

GOUREVITCH, D., "L'esthétique médicale de Galien", *LEC* 55, pp. 267-290.

GOUREVITCH, D. and GRMEK, M., "L' obésité et ses representations figures dans l'Antiquité", in V.V.A.A., *Archéologie et médecine*, pp. 355-367, Juan-les-Pins.

GREPPIN, J.A.C., "Latin nenia and the Armenian Galen dictionary", *AJPh* 108, pp. 487-490.

HANKINSON, R.J., "Causes and empiricism", *Phronesis* 32, pp. 329-348.

HARIG, G., "Bemerkungen zu Philippos", *NTM* 24.2, pp. 129-132.

— "Zur datierung der Reisen Galens. Ein Nachtrag", *Beiträge zur Hochschul und Wissenschaftgeschichte Erfurts* 21, pp. 13-20.

IERACI BIO, A.M., "Galeno e la concezione del medico", in V.V.A.A., *Talarískos: studia graeca Antonio Garzya sexagenario a discipulis oblata*, pp. 147-163, Naples.

JARCHO, S., "A history of semitertian fever", *BHM* 61, pp. 411-430.

KIBRE, P. and KELTER, I.A., "Galen's *Methodus medendi* in the Middle Ages", *HPLS* 9, pp. 17-36.

KOLLESCH, J., "Galens Auseinandersetzung mit der aristotelischen Samenlehre", in J. WIESNER (ed.), *Aristoteles: Werk und Wirkung*, pp. 17-26, Berlin.

LAÍN ENTRALGO, P., *El cuerpo humano. Oriente y Grecia antigua*. Madrid.

LOFSTEDT, B., "Zum lateinischen Kommentar von Galens Ad Glauconem", in J. HERMANN (ed.), *Latin vulgaire-Latin tardif*, pp. 145-151, Tübingen.

LÓPEZ FÉREZ, J.A., "Rheumatism, arthitris and gout in Galen", in T. APPELBOOM (ed.), *Art, history and antiquity of rheumatic diseases*, pp. 84-86, Brussels.

MARGANNE, M.H., “Un questionnaire d’anatomie”, *CE* 62, pp. 189-200.

MARMELZAT, W.L., “History of dermatologic surgery. From the beginnings to Late Antiquity”, *Clin.Dermatol* 5, pp. 1-10.

MORAUX, P., “Homère chez Galien”, in J. SERVAIS; T. HACKENS and B. SERVAIS SOYEZ (eds.), *Mélanges Labarbe*, pp. 25-37, Liege.

MORENO RODRÍGUEZ, R.Mª., “El concepto galénico de causa en la doctrina médica. Su significado en el contexto científico-social”, *Dynamis* 7-8, pp. 25-57.

NICKEL, D., *Untersuchungen zur Embryologie Galens*. Berlin.

NUTTON, V., *John Caius and the manuscripts of Galen*. Cambridge.

— “Galen’s philosophical testament “On my own opinions””, in J. WIESNER (ed.), *Aristoteles: Werk und Wirkung*, pp. 27-51, Berlin.

— “Numisianus and Galen”, *ZWG* 71, pp. 235-239.

OBERHELMAN, S.M., “The diagnostic dream in ancient medical theory and practice”, *BHM* 61, pp. 47-60.

PELLEGRIN, P., “Une oeuvre fondamentale de Galien. Essay review”, *HPLS* 9, pp. 109-114.

VIAMONTE, M., “On the Aesculapion at Pergamum; Pergamum paper; Galen and the caduceus”, *J.Fla.Med.Assoc* 74, pp. 345-348.

WILSON, N.G., “Aspects of the transmission of Galen”, in G. CAVALLO (ed.), *Le strade del resto*, pp. 45-64, Bari.

WOEHRLE, G., “Antike Bemühungen um ein System der Gerüke”, *WJA* 13, pp. 95-100.

WOODWARD, E.R., “The history of vagotomy”, *Am.J.Surg* 153, pp. 9-17.

1986

ACKERMANN, H., “Moses Maimonides (1135-1204) Ärtzliche Tätgkeit und medizinische Schriften”, *ZWG* 70, pp. 44-63.

BLAYNEY, J., “Theories of conception in the ancient Roman world”, in B. RAWSON (ed.), *The family in ancient Rome*, pp. 230-236, London.

BOYLAN, M., “Galen’s conception theory”, *JHB* 19, pp. 44-47.

BRAIN, P., *Galen on bloodletting. A Study of the Origins, Development and Validity of his Opinions*. Cambridge.

BUSH, D.C. and WILLIAMS, D.A., “Hand rehabilitation- retrospective”, *Clin.Plast.Surg* 13, pp. 293-300.

DURLING, R.J., "Burgundio of Pisa's translation of Galen's *Peri ton peponthoton topon*: *De interioribus*", *Traditio* 42, pp. 439-442.

— "Prepositional idiom in Galen", *Glotta* 64, pp. 24-30.

— "Arresting puberty", *RhM* 129, p. 364.

GAETJE, H., "Antike Lehren von Wahrnehmen bei Averroes", *ZWG* 70, pp. 129-142.

GIL SOLTRES, P., *Scripta minora de flebotomia en la tradición médica del siglo XIII*. Santander-Pamplona.

GOUREVITCH, D. and GRMEK, M.D., "*Medice, cura te ipsum*. Les maladies de Galien", *Études de lettres* 1, pp. 45-64.

HOFFMANN, Ph., "Autres données relatives à un mystérieux collaborateur d'Alde Manuce: *l'Anonymus Harvardianus*", *MEFRM* 98, pp. 675-708.

MANULI, P., "Traducibilità e molteplicità dei linguaggi nel *De placitis* di Galeno", in G. CAMBIANO (ed.), Storiografia e dossografia nella filosofia antica, pp. 245-265, Torino.

— "Le metamorfosi del femminile", in A. BARINA et. al. (eds.), *Melusina. Mito e leggenda di una donna serpente*, pp. 87-94, Roma.

MAZZINI, I., "Alimentazione e salute secondo i medici del mondo antico", *AFLM* 19, pp. 9-23.

MORENO RODRÍGUEZ, R.Mª., "Acerca de la cualidad del calor innato en las fiebres según Galeno", *Dynamis* 5-6, pp. 11-30.

PINES, S., *Studies in Arabic versions of Greek texts*. Leiden.

RAMOS CALVO, P.M.; GIORIENA de GANDARIAS, F.J. and RODRÍGUEZ BACIERO, G., "La odontología en la antigüedad. Egipto, Hipócrates, Galeno y Celso", *Rev.Esp.Estomatol* 34, pp. 427-436.

VEGETTI, M., "Tradizione e verità. Forme della storiografia filosofico-scientifica nel *De placitis* di Galeno", in G. CAMBIANO (ed.), *Storiografia e dossografia nella filosofia antica*, pp. 227-244, Torino.

WEISSER, U., "Noch einmal zur Isagoge des Johannicius. Die Herkunft des Lateneischen Lehertextes", *ZWG* 70, pp. 229-235.

WILSON, N.G., "New light on Burgundio of Pisa", *SIFC* 3, pp. 113-118.

1985

ALVERNY, M-Th., "Petro d'Albano traducteur de Galien", *Medioevo* 11, pp. 15-69.

BALDASSARRI, M., "L'introduzione alla dialettica di Galeno. Analisi e significato", in V.E. ALFIERI et al. (eds.), *Sapienza Antica: studi in onore di Domenico Pesce*, pp. 29-48, Milan.

BYLEBYL, J.J., "Medicine, philosophy and humanism in Renaissance Italy", in J.W. SHIRLEY and F.D. HONINGER (eds.), *Science and the arts in the Renaissance*, pp. 27-49, Washington.

DUDGEON, J.A., "Presentation of the Galen Medal to John Franklin Enders", *Rev.Infect.Dis* 7, pp. 278-83.

GOUREVITCH, D., "L' obésité et son traitement dans le monde romain", *History and Philosophy of the Life Sciences* 7, pp. 195-215.

GREEN, M.H., *The transmission of ancient theories of female physiology*. Princenton.

GRMEK, M.D. and GOUREVITCH, D., "Les expériences pharmacologiques dans l'antiquité", *AIHS* 35, pp. 3-27.

HOFFMANN, Ph., "Un mystérieux collaborateur d'Alde Manuce", *MEFRM* 97, pp. 45-143.

KOELBING, H.M., "Connaissances sur le cerveau", *Gesnerus* 47, pp. 315-328.

LEVET, J.P., "L'*Institutio logica* di Galeno. La syllogistique, traduction acompagnée de notes", in V.V.A.A., *D'Hippocrate à Alcuin*, pp. 57-80, Limoges.

MANETTI, D., "Tematica filosofica e scientifica nel papiro Fiorentino 115. Un probabile frammento di Galeno *In Hippocratis De Alimento*", in W. CAVINI et al. (eds.), *Studi su papiri greci di logica e medicina*, pp. 173-213, Florence.

MANULI, P., "Medico e malattia", in M. VEGETTI (ed.), *Il sapere degli antichi*, pp. 229-245, Torino.

— "L'odontoiatria nell'antichità greca e romana", in G. VOGEL and G. GAMBACORTA (eds.), *Storia dell'odontoiatria*, pp. 71-87, Milan.

MORAUX, P., *Galien de Pergame. Souvenirs d'un médecin*. Paris.

— "*Anecdota Graeca Minora*, VI. Pseudo-Galen, *De signis ex urinis*", *ZPE* 60, pp. 63-74.

MORENO RODRÍGUEZ, R.Mª., "La teoría de las discrasias y su función diagnóstica y terapeútica en la obra de Galeno", *Asclepios* 37, pp. 105-131.

MUSITELLI, S., "Da Parmenide a Galeno. Tradizioni classiche e interpretazioni medievali nelle biografie dei grandi medici antichi", *Acti Accad. Naz. Lincei. Mem. Clas. Mor. Stor. Fil.* 8.28, pp. 215-276.

NUTTON, V., "John Caius (1510-73) and the Eton Galen. Medical philology in the Renaissance", *MHJ* 20, pp. 227-252.

— "The drug trade in Antiquity", *The Journal of the Royal Society of Medicine* 78, pp. 138-145.

ORMOS, I., "Observations on Avicenna's treatise on phonetics", *AOrientHung* 39, pp. 45-84.

PEARCY, L.T., "Galen's Pergamum", *Archaeology* 38.6, pp. 33-39.

PIGEAUD, J., "Rhétorique et médicine chez les Grecs. Le cas d'Archigène", *Helmantica* 36, pp. 39-48.

— "Homo quadratus. Variations sur la beauté et la santé dans la médicine antique", *Gesnerus* 42, pp. 337-352.

— "L'humeur des anciens", *Nouvelle Revue de Psychanalyse* 32, pp. 51-69.

SCARBOROUGH, J., "Criton, physician to Trajan", in J.W. EADIE and J. OBER (eds.), *Essays in honor C.G. Starr*, pp. 387-405, Lanham.

— "Erasistratus, student of Theophrastus?", *BHM* 59, pp. 515-517.

— "Galen's dissection of the elephant", *Koroth* 8.11-12, pp. 123-134.

— "Galen on Roman amateur athletics", *Arete: The Journal of Sport Literature* 2, pp.171-176.

SCIPPERGES, H., "Galenos", in M. SCHMID (ed.), *Exempla historica. Epochen der Weltgeschichte in Biographien*, pp.189-208, Frankfurt.

TOUWAIDE, A., "Un recueil grec de pharmacologie du siècle illustré au XIV siècle. Le *Vaticanum* GR.284", *Scriptorium* 39, pp. 15-56.

TSOUYOPOULOU-SAVERIDIAU, N., "Die Zeichenlehre des Philodemos, Sextus Empirikus und Galens", in Greek Philosophical Society (ed.), *Language and reality in Greek philosophy*, pp. 235-246, Athens.

1984

BOYLAN, M., "The Galenic and Hippocratic challenges to Aristotle's conception theory", *JHB* 17, pp. 83-112.

CALAME, C., "D'Hippocrate à Galien: Trois recettes médicales sur papyrus (*P.Aberd.* 10)", *REG* 97, pp. 206-213.

CROISSANT, J., "Autour de la quatrième formule d'implication dans Sextus Empiricus (*Hyp. pyrrh.*III, 112). Essai de mise au point", *RPhA* 2.1, pp. 73-120.

DURAND, Ph., "Les oeuvres pharmacologiques de Galien. Editions et traductions latines antérieurs à (K.G.) Kühn", *CCGR* 4, pp. 75-109.

FRENCH, R.K., "An origin for the bone text of the "five-figure series"", *ZWG* 68, pp. 143-156.

GENEQUAND, C., "Quelques aspects de l'idée de nature d'Aristote à Al'Ghâzalê", *RThPh* 116, pp. 105-129.

GOUREVITCH, D., *Le triangle hippocratique dans le monde gréco-romain*. Rome.

— *Le mal d'être femme. La femme et la médecine à Rome*. Paris.

GRMEK, M., "Les vicissitudes des notions d'infection, de contagion et de germe dans la medicine antique", *Mémoires du Centre Jean Palerne* V, pp. 63-70.

HADOT, P., "Marc Aurèle était-il opiomane?", in E. LUCCHESI (ed.), *Mémoriel Festugière*, pp. 33-50, Geneve.

JOUANNA, J. and MARELLI, C., "A propos du vocabulaire hippocratique de la pathologie de l'oeil", *RPh* 58, pp. 207-215.

LINDEBOOM, G.A., "Geschichtliche Meilensteine in der Behandlung der Nachtblindheit". *CM* 19, pp. 40-49.

MACK, R.B., "From grandma to Galen: boric acid poisoning", *N.C.Med.J* 45, pp. 401-402.

MANSFELD, J., "Some Stoics on the soul (*SVF* I 136)", *Mnemosyne* 37, pp. 443-445.

MAROTH, M., "Die Stellung der Medezin", *Eirene* 21, pp. 49-57.

MUSITELLI, S., "Da Parmenide a Galeno", *MAL* 28, pp. 213-276.

NUTTON, V. "Galen in the eyes of his contemporaries", *BHM* 58, pp. 305-314.

— "From Galen to Alexander", *DOP* 38, pp. 1-14.

OTTOSSON, P.G., *Scholastic medicine and philosophy. A study of commetaries on Galen's Tegni (ca 1300-1450)*. Naples.

SCARBOROUGH, J., "Early Byzantine pharmacology", *DOP* 38, pp. 213-232.

SISSA, G., "Une virginité sans hymen. Le corps femenin en Grèce ancienne", *Annales (ESC)* 39, pp. 1111-1139.

SNOOK, G.A., "The history of sports medicine. Part I", *Am.J. Sports.Med* 12, pp. 252-254.

1983

FEHELMANN, H.R., "Ceratum Galeni. Zur Geschichte von Unguentum leniens", in P. DILG et al. (eds.), *Perspektiven der Pharmaziegeschichte. Festchrift für R. Schmitz*, pp. 65-77, Graz.

FISCHER, K.D., "Verbesserungen zur Isagoge des Johannicius", *ZWG* 67, pp. 223-224.

GILL, C., "Did Chrysippus understand Medea?", *Phronesis* 28, pp. 136-149.

GOUREVITCH, D., "Chronique anachronique, XI: Un enfant boulimique", *L'évolution psychiatrique* 48, pp. 853-857.

— "Marc Aurèle devint-il toxico-dépendant?", *L'évolution psychiatrique* 48, pp. 253-256.

GRANT, R.M., "Paul, Galen and Origin", *JThS* 34, pp. 533-536.

GRMEK, M.D., *Les maladies à l'aube de la civilisation occidentale*. Paris.

HAJAL, F., "Galen's ethical psychotherapy: its influence on a medieval Near Eastern Physician (Sinan ibn Thabit)". *JHM* 38, pp. 320-333.

KONSTANTINOU, E., "Die byzantinische Medizin im Lichte der anonymen Satire Timarion", *Byzantina* 13, pp. 159-181.

KUDLIEN, F., "Schaustellerei und Heilmittelvertrieb in der Antike", *Gesnerus* 40, pp. 91-98.

LEMAY, H.R., "Masculinity and feminity in early Renaissance treatises on human reproduction", *CM* 18, pp. 21-31.

MANULI, P., "Lo stile del commento. Galeno e la tradizione ippocratica", in G. GIANNANTONI and M. VEGETTI (eds.), *La scienza ellenistica*, pp. 375-394, Naples.

— "Donne mascoline, femmine sterili, vergini perpetue. La ginecologia greca tra Ippocrate e Sorano", in S. CAMPESE; P. MANULI AND G. SISSA (eds.), *Madre materia*, pp. 149-192, Torino.

MORAUX, P., "Ein unbekannter Lehrer Galens", *ZPE* 53, pp. 85-88.

MORENO RODRIGUEZ, R.Mª., "El concepto de diáthesis παρὰ φύσιν (estado preternatural) en la patología de Galeno", *Dynamis* 3, pp. 7-27.

NUTTON, V., "The beneficial ideology", *Chiron* 14, pp. 209-222.

OBERHELMAN, S.M., "Galen, *On Diagnosis from Dreams*", *JHM* 38, pp. 36-47.

OTIS, A.B., "A perspective of respiratory mechanics", *J.Appl.Physiol.* 54, pp. 1183-1187.

PEARCY, L.T., "Galen and the Stoic rhetoric", *GRBS* 24, pp. 259-272.

ROUSSELLE, A., "Parole et inspiration. Le travail de la voix dans le monde romain", *HPLS* 5, pp. 129-157.

WEISSER, U., "Thabit ibn Qurra's Epitome of Galen's book on seventh-month children", *JHAS* 7, pp. 141-144.

1982

ALSINA, J., *Los orígenes helénicos de la medicina occidental*. Barcelona.

BRAIN, P., *Galen's pathology. Concepts and contradictions*. Durban.

DAVIES, J.W., "Prompt cooling of burned areas: a review of benefits and the effector mechanisms", *Burns.Incl.Therm.Inj*. 9, pp. 1-6.

DURLING, R.J., "Lexicographical notes on Galen's writings, (Part III)", *Glotta* 60, pp. 236-244.

FACAL, J.L. and GONZÁLEZ, A., *Repertorium litterarum ex codicibus, papyris epigraphis*. Madrid.

FITZGERALD, F.T., "From Galen to Xerox: the authoritarian reference in medicine". *Ann.Intern.Med* 96, pp. 245-246.

GOUREVITCH, D., "Médecins fous", *L'évolution psychiatrique* 47, pp. 1113-1118.

GREPPIN, J.A.C., "Preliminary comments on the Greek-Armenian lexicon to Galen", *REArm* 16, pp. 69-80.

LEDEN, H., "Laryngology: from Galen to García", *Otolaryngol.Head.Neck.Surg*. 90, pp. 226-232.

MARKETOS, S.G. and BALLAS, C.N., "Bronchial asthma in the medical literature of Greek antiquity", *J.Asthma* 19, pp. 263-269.

MORENO RODRÍGUEZ, R.Mª. and GARCÍA BALLESTER, L., "El dolor en la teoría y práctica médica de Galeno", *Dynamis* 2, pp. 3-24.

MOSZYNSKI, J., "Galenus: *De victu attenuante*", *Arch.Hist.Med. Warsz* 45, pp. 61-75.

NABIELEK, R., "Probleme bei der Edition der nur arabisch überlilieferten pseudogalenischen Schrift *De somno et vigilia*", *NTM* 19.2, pp. 75-80.

RENGER, F.G., "Zur Geschichte der Hepatologie von Galen bis Frerichs", *Dtsch.Z.Verdau.Stoffwechselkr* 42, pp. 193-202.

SHARPLES, R.W., "Alexander. On time", *Phronesis* 27, pp. 55-81.

TSOUKANELIS, A., "Concerning Archigenes and Galen: correcting an historical error", *Bull.Hist.Dent*. 36, pp. 87-90.

1981

BAADER, G., "Galen im mittelalterlichen Abendland", in V. NUTTON (ed.), *Galen: problems and prospects*, pp. 213-228, London.

DEGEN, R., "Galen im Syrischen. Eine Übersicht über die syrische überlieferung der Werke Galens", in V. NUTTON (ed.), *Galen: problems and prospects*, pp. 131-136, London.

DURLING, R.J., "Lexicographical notes on Galen's writings (Part II)", *Glotta* 59, pp. 108-116.

— "*Corrigenda* and *addenda* to Diels' *Galenica*", *Traditio* 37, pp. 373-381.

EASTWOOD, B.S., "Galen on the elements of olfactory sensation", *RhM* 124, pp. 268-290.

FREDE, M., "On Galen's epistemology", in V. NUTTON (ed.), *Galen: problems and prospects*, pp. 65-86, London.

GARCÍA BALLESTER, L., "Experiencia y especulación en el diagnóstico galénico", *Dynamis* 1, pp. 203-223.

— "Galen as a medical practitioner; problems in diagnosis", in V. NUTTON (ed.), *Galen: problems and prospects*, pp. 13-46, London.

GAROFALO, I., "Le Anatomikal Enkheiréseis di Galeno e la traduzione araba della scuola di Hunain Ibn Ishaq", *SCO* 31, pp. 257-277.

GOUREVITCH, D., "Simulation", *L'évolution psychiatrique* 46, pp. 205-209.

HALLEUX, R., "Une description pseudo-aristotélicienne de mines de Chypre", *AC* 50, pp. 382-392.

JOHNSTONE, P., "Galen in Arabic; the transformation of Galenic pharmacology", in V. NUTTON (ed.), *Galen: problems and prospects*, pp. 197-212, London.

KOLLESCH, J., "Galen und die Zweite Sophistik", in V. NUTTON (ed.), *Galen: problems and prospects*, pp. 1-12, London.

KUDLIEN, F., "Galen's religious belief", in V. NUTTON (ed.), *Galen: problems and prospects*, pp. 117-130, London.

LIEBER, E., "Galen in Hebrew; the transmission of Galen's works in the medieval Islamic world", in V. NUTTON (ed.), *Galen: problems and prospects*, pp. 167-186, London.

MANETTI, D., "Un nuovo papiro di Galeno. P. Mon. Gr. Inv. 329: *De placitis* I (88,20-31; 90,11-20 DeLacy)", *Studi di lett. Greca* 1, pp. 115-123.

MORAUX, P., "Galien comme philosophe; la philosophie de la nature", in V. NUTTON (ed.), *Galen: problems and prospects*, pp. 87-116, London.

NUTTON, V. (ed.), *Galen: problems and prospects*. London.

PALMIERI, N., "Un antico commento a Galeno della scuola medica di Ravenna", *Physis* 23, pp. 197-296.

PETERSEN, E.S., "Galen: the most maligned physician", *Proc. Inst.Med.Chic.* 34, p. 12.

PREUS, A., "Intention and impulse in Aristotle and the Stoics", *Apeiron* 15, pp. 48-58.

ROSNER, F., "The medical writings of Maimonides", *CM* 16, pp. 1-11.

SCARBOROUGH, J., "The Galenic question", *ZWG* 65, pp. 1-31.

STROHMAIER, G., "Galen in Arabic; prospects and projects", in V. NUTTON (ed.), *Galen: problems and prospects*, pp. 187-196, London.

VEGETTI, M., "Modelli di medicina in Galeno", in V. NUTTON (ed.), *Galen: problems and prospects*, pp. 47-64, London.

WEAR, A., "Galen in the Rennaissance", in V. NUTTON (ed.), *Galen: problems and prospects*, pp. 229-262, London.

WILKIE, J.S. and LLOYD, G.E.R., "The Arabic version of Galen's *Ars parva*", *JHS* 101, pp. 145-148.

1980

BURGUIERE, P. and JACQUES, J.M., *Galien témoin des pharmacologues anciens*. Bordeaux.

DONINI, P., "Motivi filosofici in Galeno", *La Parola del Passato* 35, pp. 333-370.

DURLING, R.J., "Lexicographical notes on Galen's writings (Part I)", *Glotta* 58, pp. 260-266.

EASTWOOD, B.S., "Cosmology and physiology in Galenic visual theory: Hunayn Ibn Ishaq", *Trans.Stud.Coll.Physicians.Phila* 2, pp. 276-283.

ESPINOSA, P., "La *téchne iatriké* de Galeno: problemática de una traducción a idioma moderno", in S. GARMA PONS (ed.), *El científico español ante su historia: la ciencia en España entre 1750-1850*, pp. 553-563, Madrid.

HAU, F.R., "Die Bildung des Arxtes im islamischen Mittelalter", *CM*, pp. 7-33.

JACKSON, R., *Doctors and Diseases in the Roman Empire*. London.

JOUANNA, J. and TAILLARDAT, J., "Une vox nihili: *Fereatikôs* dans le glossaire hippocratique de Galien (Kühn XIX 151,3), *REG* 93, pp. 126-135.

MANETTI, D., "Una glossa ippocratica di Galeno", *Athenaeum* 58, pp. 462-465.

MANULI, P., "Fisiologia e patologia del femminile negli scritti ippocratici dell'antica ginecologia greca", in CNRS (ed.), *Hippocratica. Actes du Colloque hippocratique de Paris*, pp. 393-408, Paris.

— *Medicina e antropologia nella tradizione antica*. Torino.

MARGANNE, M.H., "Une étape dans la transmission d'une prescription médicale: P.Berl.Möller 13", in R. PINTAUDI (ed.), *Miscellanea Papyrologica*, pp. 179-183, Florence.

PEROSA, A., "Codici dc Galeno postillati dal Poliziano", in P.O. KRISTELLER et al. (eds.), *Umanesimo e rinascimento*, pp. 75-109, Florence.

ROUSSELLE, A., "Le corps de la femme d'après les médecins grecs", *Annales (ESC)* 35, pp. 1089-1115.

THOMASEN, A.L., "*Historia animalium*" contra "*Gynaecia*" in der Literatur des Mittelalters", *CM* 15, pp. 5-24.

VEGETTI, M., "La polemica di Galeno contro la medicina metodica", *SicGymn* 33, pp. 427-435.

WINKLER, L., *Galens Schrift De antidotis. Ein Beitrag zur Geschichte von Antidot und Theriak*. Marburg.

1979

BARIGAZZI, A., "Sul titolo del *Protrettico* di Galeno", *Prometheus* 5, pp. 157-163.

BRINK, A., "Depression and loss: a theme in Robert Burton's "Anatomy of melancholy" (1621)", *Can.J.Psychiatry* 24, pp. 767-772.

BYLEBYL, J.J., "The medical side of Harvey's discovery: the normal and the abnormal", *Henry.E.Sigerist.Suppl.BHM* 2, pp. 28-102.

DE LACY, Ph., "Galen's concept of continuity", *GRBS* 20, pp. 355-369.

FRENCH, R.K., "De *Juvamentis Membrorum* and the reception of Galenic physiological anatomy", *Isis* 70, pp. 96-109.

GARCÍA BALLESTER, L., "Studies on Hippocrates and Galen in modern Spain", *Trans.Stud.Coll.Physicians.Phila*, 1, pp. 215-29.

JOUANNA, J., "Une forme étymologique retrouvée dans le glossaire hippocratique de Galien", *RPh* 53, pp. 260-262.

KOTRC., R.F. and WALTERS, K.R., "A bibliography of the Galenic Corpus. A newly researched list and arrangement of the titles of the treatises extant in Greek, Latin, and Arabic", *Trans. and Stud. of the College of Physicians of Philadelphia* 1, pp. 256-304.

LIEBER, E., "Galen: physician as philosopher; Maimonides: philosopher as physician", *BHM* 53, pp. 268-285.

MACLEOD, M.D., "Lucian's activities as a μισαλάζων", *Philologus* 123, pp. 326-328.

MAROTH, M., "Galenos und die vierte Figur der Syllogismen", *AAntHung* 27, pp. 187-205.

SIDER, D. and McVAUGH, M., "Galen on tremor, palpitation, spasm, and rigor", *Trans.Stud.Coll.Physicians.Phila* 1, pp. 183-210.

SMITH, W.D., *The Hippocratic Tradition.* Ithaca-London.

SNOOK, G.A., "The father of sports medicine (Galen)", *Am.J. Sports.Med* 6, pp. 128-131.

STROHMAIER, G., "Ärtztliche Ausbildung im islamischen Mittelalter", *Klio* 61, pp. 519-524.

ULLMANN, M., "Die arabische Überlieferung der Werke des Rufus von Ephesos", in Y. AHMAD et al. (eds.) *Proceedings of the First International Symposium for the History of Arabic Science* II, pp. 348-357, Aleppo.

WEISSER, U., "Die hippokratische Lehre von den Siebenmonatskindern bei Galen und Tabit ibn Qurra", *ZWG* 63, pp. 209-238.

ZORGNIOTTI, A.W., "Galenic urology: translation of urologic portions of *De Locis Affectis* (Book VI, Chapter 3): Part II", *Urology* 13, pp. 701-703.

1978

BARIGAZZI, A., "Solone, Saffo, Euripide in un passo di Galeno", *Prometheus* 4, pp. 207-218.

FRENCH, R.K. and LLOYD, G.E.R., "Greek fragments of the lost books of Galen's *Anatomical Procedures*", *ZWG* 62, pp. 235-249.

GUGGENHEIMER, E.H., "Talmudic evidence for Greek spelling", *SicGymn* 31, pp. 313-314.

KOTTEK, S.S., "The seat of the soul", *CM* 13, pp. 219-246.

KUDLIEN, F., "Medicinische Aspekte der antiken Unsterblichkeitvorstellung", *RhM* 121, pp. 218-225.

KURDZIALEK., "Die psychosomatischen Bedingungen sittlicher Laster", *ZWG* 62, pp. 175-189.

LYTTON, D.G. and RESURHR, L,M., "Galen on abnormal swellings", *JHM* 33, pp. 531-549.

MAURACH, G., "Johannicius. Isagoge as Techne Galeni", *ZWG* 62, pp. 148-174.

RADBILL, S.X., "Pediatric dermatology in antiquity: part III", *Int.J.Dermatol* 17, pp. 427-434.

SCHIPPERGES, H., "Antike und Mittelalter", in H. SCHIPPERGES et al. (eds.), *Krankheit, Heilkunst, Heilung*, pp. 229-269, Freiburg.

SCHMITH, V., "Ein vermutetes Epicharm-Fragment bei Galen", *LZPE* 30, pp. 13-17.

WILKIE, J.S. and LLOYD, G.E.R., "The Arabic version of Galen's *De sectis ad eos qui introducuntur*", *JHS* 98, pp. 167-169.

WILSON, N.G., "A Byzantine miscellany", *JOEByz* 27, pp. 157-179.

1977

BRAIN, P., "Galen on the Ideal of the Physician", *South African Medical Journ.* 51, pp. 936-938.

BRUNNER, F.G., *Pathologie und Therapie der Geschwülzte in der antiken Medizin bei Celsus und Galen*. Zürich.

BYLEBYL, J.J., "Nutrition, quantification and circulation", *BHM* 51, pp. 369-385.

DILLON, J., *The middle Platonists. A study of platonism (80 B.C. to A.D.220)*. London.

FORMENTIN, M., "Galenus. *De anatomia internarum et externarum partium*", *AFLPad* 2, pp. 83-92.

GUIDORIZZI, G., "Nota a Galeno, *Quomodo simulantes sint deprehendendi* (XIX, 1 K)", *RFIC* 105, pp. 157-161.

HARIG, G., "Die antike Auffassung vom Gift", *NTM* 14, pp. 104-112.

INGENKAMP, H.G., "Introspektion in der naturwissenschaftlichen Psychologie", *RhM* 120, pp. 30-44.

KONSTANTINIDES, M.Z., *The Greek manuscripts of Galeni De tremore, palpitatione, convulsione et rigore liber, with a critical edition of chapters 1-5*. New York.

KOTCR, R.F., "A new fragment of Erasistratus", *RhM* 120, pp. 159-161.

MANULI, P., "La techne medica nella tradizione encefalocentrica e cardio-emocentrica", in R. JOLY (ed.), *Corpus Hippocraticum. Actes du Colloque hippocratique de Mons*, pp. 183-195, Mons.

— "Cuore, sangue e cervello da Alcmeone ad Aristotele. Con Appendice su Galeno e l'antropologia platonica", in P. MANULI and M. VEGETTI (eds.), *Cuore, sangue et cervello. Biologia e antropologia nel pensiero antico*, pp. 29-195, Milan.

MANULI, P. and VEGETTI, M. (eds.), *Cuore, sangue et cervello. Biologia e antropologia nel pensiero antico*. Milan.

MORAUX, P., "Unbekannte Galen-Scholien", *ZPE* 27, pp. 1-63.

NUTTON, V., "A forgotten manuscript of Galenus Latinus", in J.DUMMER and K. TREU (eds.), *Studia Codicologica*, pp. 331-340, Berlin.

— "Archiatri and the medical profession in Antiquity", *Papers of the British School at Rome* 45, pp. 191-226.

PENELLA, R.J., "Galen, *De bono habitu* 752 K", *RhM* 120, pp. 166-167.

PETERSON, D.W., "Observations on the chronologie of the Galenic corpus", *BHM* 51, pp. 484-495.

PREUS, A., "Galen's criticism of Aristotle's conception theory", *JHB* 10, pp. 65-85.

SEIFERT, A., "Historia im Mittelalter", *ABG* 21, pp. 226-284.

STROHMAIER, G., "Galen über die Vereinsamung des Menschen in der Gross-stadt", *FBSM* 18, pp. 197-198.

TODD, R.B., "Galenic medical ideas in the Greek Aristotelian commentators", *SO* 52, pp. 117-134.

— "The author of the *De qualitatibus incorporeis*", *AC* 46, pp. 198-204.

ULLMANN, M., "Zwei spätantike Kommentare zur hippocratischen Schrift *De morbis mulieribus*", *MHJ* 12, pp. 245-262.

— "Galenus Kommentar zur der Schrift *De aere aquis locis*", in R. JOLY (ed.), *Corpus Hippocraticum. Actes du Colloque hippocratique de Mons*, pp. 353-365, Mons.

VILLEY, R., "La médicine latine, Galien, II", in J. POULET; J.C. SOURNIA and M. MARTINY (eds.), *Histoire de la médicine, de la pharmacie, d'art dentaire et de l'art véterinaire*, pp. 11-39, Paris.

1976

ANNA, M., "La diagnosi in odontostomatologia dalle tavolette babilonesi alle collezioni Ippocratiche e di Galeno", *Dent. Cadmos* 44, pp. 53-54.

BALTES, M., *Die Weltentstehung des platonischen Timaios nach den antichen Interpreten*. Leiden.

BARNARD, L.W., "Athenagoras, *De resurrectione*. The background and theology of a second century *On the resurrection*", *STh* 30, pp. 1-42.

CHIARI, A., "Matro, Conv. Att. 27-32", *Sileno* 2, pp. 328-330.

ESPINOSA, P., "Anotaciones a la *Téchne iatriké* de Galeno", *Asclepios* 18, pp. 235-242.

FROST, E.A., "Tracing the tracheostomy", *Ann.Otol.Rhinol. Laryngol* 85, pp. 618-624.

HARIG, G., "Der Begriff der lauen Wärme in der theoretischen Pharmakologie zwischen Medizin und Mathematik in der Antike", *NTM* 13, pp. 70-76.

JOBE, T.H., "Medical theories of melancholia in the seventeenth and early eigthteenth centuries", *CM* 11, pp. 217-231.

JOUANNA, J., "Le traité hippocratique *Des affections internes* (c.35) et le Glossaire hippocratique de Galien. A propos des plantes denommées "chore, choris" et "chorion", *RPh* 50, pp. 32-40.

— "Le traité *Du régime des maladies aiguës*", *RHT* 6, pp. 1-30.

MANULI, P., "Il dibattito sulla medicina nel V secolo", in M. VEGETTI (ed.), *Opere di Ippocrate*, pp. 125-139, Torino.

MARINONE, N., "Galeno. *De victu attenuante* 78 e 98", *RFIC* 104, pp. 328-336.

MOES, R.J., "Andreas Vesalius and the anatomy of the upper extremity", *J.Hand.Surg.Am* 1, pp. 23-28.

MORAUX, P., "Galien et Aristote", in F. BOSSIER et al. (eds.), *Images of man in ancient and medieval thought. Studia Verbeke ab amicis et collegis dicata*, pp. 127-146, Leuven.

NICKEL, D., "Ein Ballspiel im Urteit des Arztes. Bemerkungen zu Galens Schrift Üver die Übung mit dem kleinen Ball", *NTM* 13, pp. 77-81.

SCARBOROUGH, J., "Galen's investigations of the kidney", *CM* 11, pp. 171-177.

STROHMAIER, G., "Übersehenes zur Biographie Lukians", *Philologus* 120, pp. 117-122.

THESAURUS LINGUAE GRAECAE. *A Bibliography of the Greek Medical Writers*. Berkeley.

TRACY, T.J., "Plato, Galen and the center of conciousness", *ICS* 1, pp. 43-52.

VIRIEUX-REIMOND, A., *Pour connaître la pensée des Stoïciens*. Paris.

YOUTIE, L.C., “A medical prescription for an eye-salve”, *ZPE* 23, pp. 121-129.

ZIMMERMANN, F.W., “Al-Farabi und die philosophische Kritik an Galen von Alexander zu Averroes”, in *Akten des VII Kongr. für Arabistik und Islamwiss*, pp. 401-414, Göttingen.

1975

AFRICA, T.W., “Archimedes through the looking-glass”, *CW* 68, pp. 305-308.

BLEKER, J., “Zur Physiologie und Pathologie der Nieren bei Galen”, *ZWG* 59, pp. 321-327.

BULL, J.W., “The nervous system’s blood vessels from Galen to Rontgen and after”, *Proc.R.Soc.Med* 68, pp. 695-702.

CARDONA, G., “Tolomeo e Galeno”, in M. del PARA (ed.), *La filosofia ellenistica e la patristica christiana dal III secolo a.C. al V secolo d.C.*, pp. 229-249, Milan.

CIUFFREDA, K.J. and STARK, L., “Descartes’ law of reciprocal innervation”, *Am.J.Optom.Physiol.Opt*, 52, pp. 663-673.

GAROFALO, I., “Due passi del *De Experientia medica* di Galeno”, *ASNP* 5, pp. 1305-1306.

GOUREVITCH, D., “A propos de la simulation dans l’antiquité. Galien et sa monographie princeps *Quomodo morbum simulantes sint deprehendi libellus*”, *Méd.lég.exp.méd* 1, pp. 13-18.

HARIG, G. and KOLLESCH, J., “Galen und Hippocrates”, in Université des sciences humaines de Strasbourg. Centre de recherches sur la Grèce antique (ed.), *La Collection hippocratique et son rôle dans l’histoire de la médecine*, pp.257-274, Leiden.

KEIL, G.; MOKHTAR, A.M. and THIES, H.J., “Galenkritik bei Rhazes. Zur Wertung der Autoritatskritik im islamischen Mittelalter”, *Med.Monatsschr* 25, pp. 559-563.

MANSFELD, J., “Alcmacon physikós or physician? With some remarks on Calcidius’ *On vision compared to Galen’s Plac. Hippo. Plat. VII*”, in J. MANSFELD and L.M. DE RIJK (eds.), *Kephalaion: studies in Greek Philosophy and its continuation offered to Prof. C.J. Vogel*, pp. 26-38, Assen.

MAROTH, M., “Die Eisagoge bei den Araben”, *ZAnt* 25, pp. 457-460.

MOLINA-NEGRO, P. and HARDY, J., “Semiology of Tremors”, *Can. J.Neurol.Sci*, 2, pp. 23-29.

POST, C.J. and SCARBOROUGH, J., “On Ballester’s Galen. An extended review”, *Episteme* 9, pp. 3-31.

REEDY, J., “Galen on cancer and related diseases”, *CM* 10, pp. 227-238.

SCARBOROUGH, J., "The drug lore of Asclepiades of Bithinia", *Pharmacy in History* 17, pp. 43-57.

SIEGEL, R.E., *Galen's system of physiology and medicine.* Basel.

— "Aristotle's and Galen's doctrines of respiration and blood flow", *Episteme* 9, pp. 171-188.

TOBIN, R., "The canon of Polykleitos", *AJA* 79, pp. 307-321.

TOOMER, G.J., "Galen on the astronomers and astrologers", *AHES* 32, pp. 193-206.

ULLMANN, M., "Die Schrift des Rufus *De infantium curatione* und das Problem der *Autorenlemmata* in der *Collectiones medicae* des Oribasius", *MHJ* 10, pp. 165-190.

WASSERSTEIN, A., "Aqua Damnata", *Hermes* 103, pp. 382-383.

1974

ALSINA, J., "Deux notes hippocratiques", *StudClas* 16, pp. 211-216.

DILLER, H., "Empirie und Logos Galens Stellung zu Hippokrates und Platon". in K. DÖRING and W. KULLMANN (eds.), *Studia Platonica, Festschr. H. Gundert,* pp. 227-238, Amsterdam.

GARCÍA BALLESTER, L., "Diseases of the soul in Galen. The impossibility of a Galenic psychotherapy", *CM* 9, pp. 35-43.

GRACIA, D. and VIDAL, J.L., "La *Isagoge* de Ioannitius. Introducción, edición, traducción y notas", *Asclepios* 26-27, pp. 267-382.

GROSS, K., "Galens teleologische Betractung der menschlichen Hand in *De usu partium*", *ZWG* 58, pp. 13-24.

HALL, T.S., "Greek medical and philosophical interpretations of fear", *Bull.N.Y.Acad.Med.* 50, pp. 821-832.

HARIG, G., *Bestimmung der Intensitat im medizinischen System Galens. Beitrag zur theoretischen Pharmacologie, Nosologie und Therapie in der galenischen Medizin.* Berlin.

LACKNER, W., "Eine Konjektur zur Lücke in Ciceros *De nat. deor*. II, 137", *GB* 2, pp. 93-96.

PETERSON, M.D., *Galen's Therapeutics to Glaucon and its early commentaires.* Baltimore.

STROHMAIER, G., "Hunayn ben Ishaq et le serment hippocratique", *Arabica* 21, pp. 318-323.

TOLEDO-PEREYRA, L.H., “A surgeon of antiquity”, *Surg.Gynecol. Obstet* 138, pp. 767-770.

1973

GUIDORIZZI, G., “L’opusculo di Galeno *De dignotione ex insomnis*”, *BPEC* 21, pp. 81-105.

HARRIS, C.R.S., *The heart and vascular system From Alcmaeon to Galen*. Oxford.

KOLLESCH, J., *Untersuchungen zu pseudo-galenischen Definitiones medicae*. Berlin.

KOTRC, R.F., “Critical notes on Galen’s *De venae sectione adversus Erasistrateos Romae degentes* (K. XI, 197-249)”, *CQ* 23, pp. 369-374.

KUDLIEN, F., “Empirie und Theorie in der Harnlehere des Johannes Aktuarios”, *CM* 8, pp. 19-30.

LITTMAN, R.J. and LITTMAN, M.L., “Galen and the Antonine plague”, *AJPh* 94, pp. 243-255.

NUTTON, V., “The chronology of Galen’s early career”, *CQ* 23, pp. 158-171.

— “Sextus or Commodus”, *Chiron* 3, pp. 424-437.

OGDEN, M.S., “The Galenic works cited in Guy de Chauliac’s *Chirurgia magna*”, *JHM* 28 pp. 24-33.

SHAPIRO, S.L., “The skeptical anatomist (Galen), (Vesalius)”, *Eye.Ear.Nose.Throat.Mon.* 51, pp. 103-107.

SIEGEL, R.E., *Galen on psychology, psychopathology and function and diseases of the nervous systems. And analysis of this doctrines, observations and experiments*. Basel.

SMITH, W.D., “Galen on Coans versus Cnidians”, *BHM* 47, pp. 569-585.

SOLMSEN, F., “Early Christian interest in the theory of demostration”, in W. den BOER (ed.), *Romanitas et Christianitas; studia Iano Henrico Waszink,* pp. 281-291, Amsterdam

TEMKIN, O., *Galenism: rise and decline of a medical philosophy*. New York.

TOLEDO-PEREYRA, L.H., “Galen’s contribution to surgery”, *JHM* 28, pp. 357-375.

1972

BARNARD, L.W., “Galen, Marcus Aurelius and Celsus”, *Theol. Hist* 18, pp. 53-68.

BIRLEY, A.R., “A nickname for Commodus and the date of Fronto’s death”, *Chiron* 2, pp. 463-473.

DE LACY, Ph., "Galen's Platonism", *AJPh* 93, pp. 27-39.

FABRICIUS, C., *Galens Excerpte aus älteren Pharmakologen*. Berlin.

FURLEY, D.J. and WILKIE, J.S., "An Arabic translation solves some problems in Galen", *CR* 22, pp. 164-167.

GARCÍA BALLESTER, L., *Alma y enfermedad en la obra de* Galeno. Madrid.

— *Galeno en la sociedad y en la ciencia de su tiempo*. Madrid.

KIDD, I.G., "Posidonius on emotions", in A.A. LONG (ed.), *Problems in Stoicism*, pp. 200-215, London.

KUDLIEN, F. and WILSON, N.G., "Galen", in C.C. GILLISPIE (ed.), *Dictionary of Scientific biography*, vol. 5, pp. 227-237, New York.

LAÍN ENTRALGO, P. (ed.), *Historia Universal de la Medicina*. Barcelona.

NUTTON, V., "Galen and the medical autobiography", *PcPhS* 18, pp. 50-62.

PAGEL, W., "Peripheral venous flow ascending to the heart (Ficinus 1489) and the spread of poison", *Episteme* 6, pp. 128-134.

RENCHAN, R., "The Greek philosophical background of Fourt Maccabees", *RhM* 115, pp. 223-238.

RODNAN, G.P. and BENEDEK, T.G., "Hippocrates, Galen, and synovia", *Ann.Intern.Med* 76, pp. 834-835.

SIEGEL, R.E., "Galen's concept of blood letting in relation to his ideas on pulmonary and peripheral blood flood and blood formation", in A.G. DEBUS (ed.) *Science, medicine and society in the Renaissance; essays in honor of Walter Pagel*, pp. 243-275, New York.

TAYLOR, F.K., "Sydenham's disease entities", *Psychol.Med* 12, pp. 243-250.

TEMKIN, O., *The falling Sickness: history of epilepsy from the Greeks to the Beginnings of modern neurology*. Baltimore.

WALSH, J., "Galen visits the Dead Sea and the copper mines of Cyprus", *Bulletin of the Geographical Society of Philadelphia* 25, pp. 93-110.

1971

BENEDUM, J., "Statilos Attalos. Ein Beitrage medizinhistorische Numismatik der Antike", *MHJ* 6, p. 264-277.

BYLEBYL, J.J., "Galen on the non-natural causes of variation in the pulse", *BHM* 45, pp. 482-485.

BYLEBYL, J.J. and PAGEL, W., "The chequered career of Galen's doctrine on the pulmonary veins", *Med.Hist* 15, pp. 211-229.

DONINI, P., "L'anima e gli elementi nel *De Anima* di Alessandro di Afrodisia", *AAT* 105, pp. 61-107.

GAERTNER, H., "Eine Kallianax- Anakdote bei Galen und Palladios", *Hermes* 99, pp. 243-246.

GARCÍA BALLESTER, L., "Aproximación genética a la obra anatómica de Galeno", *Asclepios* 23, pp. 191-209.

— "La utilización de Platón y Aristóteles en los escritos tardíos de Galeno", *Episteme* 5, pp. 112-120.

KUDLIEN, F., "Galens Urteil über die Thukydideische Pestenbeschreibung", *Episteme* 5, pp. 132-133.

MARINONE, N., "Ghiande e castagne in un emendamento a Galeno", *RFIC* 99, pp. 435-440.

McVAUGH, M.R. and MAUSSKOPF, S.H., "A Galenic model for quantitative physiological reasoning: a further note", *BHM* 45, pp. 179-180.

NIEBYL, P.H., "Old age, fever, and the lamp metaphor", *JHM* 26, pp. 351-368.

— "The non-natural causes", *BHM* 45, pp. 486-492.

RATHER, L.J., "Disturbance of function (functio laesa): the legendary fifth cardinal sign of inflammation, added by Galen to the four cardinal signs of Celsus", *Bull.N.Y.Acad.Med.* 47, pp. 303-322.

SCARBOROUGH, J., "Galen and the gladiators", *Episteme* 5, pp. 98-110.

SIEGEL, R.E., "Galen on the innervation and neurophysiology of the 17th and 18th centuries", *Episteme* 5, pp. 121-131.

SMITH, E.S., "Galen's account of the cranial nerves and the autonomic nervous system. 1", *CM* 6, pp. 77-98.

— "Galen's account of the cranial nerves and the autonomic nervous system. 2", *CM* 6, pp. 173-194.

1970

ALEXANDERSON, B., "Bemerkungen zu Galens Com. Nat. hom., Comm. acut., *De temperamentis* und *De placitis*", *Eranos* 68, pp. 61-75.

BORLONE, E., "Perché la dottrina anatomo-phisiologica post-aristotelica invento la porositá del setto?", *PSM* 20, pp. 92-102.

DAVIES, J.C., "Galen and arteries", *Br.Med.J* 1, pp. 567-568.

DOBY, T., "Vascular experiments before Harvey", *Episteme* 4, pp. 146-156.

JARCHO, S., "Galen's six non-naturals: a bibliographic note and translation", *BHM* 44, pp. 372-377.

LAÍN ENTRALGO, P., *La medicina hipocrática*. Madrid.

LIEBER, E., "Galen on contaminated cereals as a cause of epidemics", *BHM* 44, pp. 332-345.

MAY, M.T., "On translating Galen", *JHM* 25, pp. 168-176.

NUTTON, V., "Prognostica Galieni", *Med.Hist.* 14, pp. 96-100.

SIEGEL, R.E., *Galen on sense perception. His doctrines, observations and experiments on vision, hearing, smell, taste, touch and pain, and their historical sources*. Basel.

— "Principles and contradictions of Galen's doctrine of vision", *ZWG* 54, pp. 261-276.

— "Galen on surgery of the pericardium: an early record of therapy based on anatomic and experimental studies", *Am.J. Cardiol* 26, pp. 524-527.

WINDEN, J.C.M., "Le christianisme et la Philosophie. Le commencement du dialogue entre la foi et la raison, I", in P. GRANFIELD and J.A. JUNGMANN (eds.), *Kyriakon. Festschrift Johannes Quasten*, pp. 205-213, Münster.

1969

BOWERSOCK, G.B., *Greek sophists in the Roman Empire*. Oxford.

GARCÍA BALLESTER, L., "La psyché en el somaticismo médico de la Antigüedad. La actitud de Galeno", *Episteme* 3, pp. 195-209.

GIL, L., *Therapeia. La medicina popular en el mundo clásico*. Madrid.

HENSCHEN, F., "On the term diabetes in the works of Aretaeus and Galen", *Med.Hist* 13, pp. 190-192.

LIND, L.R., "A new manuscript fragment of Constantine Africanus Compendium Megatechni Galeni", in B.E. PERRY (ed.), *Classical Studies presented to B. Perry by his students and colleagues at the University of Illinois*, pp. 103-113, Illinois.

LOPEZ PIÑERO, J.M. and MORALES, J.M., *Neurosis y psicoterapia. Un estudio histórico*. Madrid.

NIKITAS, A., "Textkritische Bemerkungen zum zwiten Epidemienbuch des Corpus Hippocraticum", *Hermes* 97, pp. 187-197.

NISHIKAWA, A., "Sensation and thought in Demokritus", *JCS* 17, pp. 28-38.

NUTTON, V., “The doctor and the oracle”, *RBPh* 47, pp. 37-48.

PAZZINI, A., “Il concetto di umanesimo nella storia della medicina”, *PSM* 19.5, pp. 5-17.

SCARBOROUGH, J., “The classical of the Vesalian revolution”, *Episteme* 2, pp. 200-218.

SIEGEL, R.E., “Did the Greek atomists considerer a non-corpuscular visual transmission? Reconsideration of some ancient visual doctrines”, *AIHS* 22, pp. 3-16.

1968

AMERIO, A., “Galeno puericultore. Nota preliminare”, *PSM* 22.5, pp. 24-27.

COTURRI, E., “Il ritrovamento di antichi testi di medicina nel primo secolo del Rinascimiento”, *Episteme* 2, pp. 91-110.

DURLING, R.J., “*Lectiones Galenicae. Téchne iatriké*. Kühn I, 305-412”, *CPH* 63, pp. 56-57.

FERRARI, G., “Su una recente traduzione dell’opera *Institutio logica* di Galeno”, *Episteme* 2, pp. 244-248.

GARCÍA BALLESTER, L., “Lo médico y lo filosófico-moral en las relaciones entre alma y enfermedad”, *Asclepio* 20, pp. 22-28.

— “El hipocratismo de Galeno”, *Bol.Soc.Esp.His.Med.* 8, pp. 22-28.

— *Alma y enfermedad en la obra de Galeno*. Valencia.

GRENSEMANN, H., “Weitere Bemerkungen zu den Hippokratesglossaren des Erotian und Galen”, *Hermes* 96, pp. 177-190.

KUDLIEN, F., “Antike Anatomie und menschlicher Leichnam”, *Hermes* 3, pp. 305-336.

— “The third century A.D. A blank spot in the history of medicine?”, in O. TEMKIN et al. (eds.), *Medicine, science and culture. Historical essays in Honor of O. Temkin*, pp. 25-34, Baltimore.

MARTINI, U. de., “L’isterismo da Ippocrate a Charcot”, *PSM* 12, pp. 42-49.

MUSITELLI, S., “Riflessi di teorie mediche nelle *Baccanti* di Euripide”, *Dioniso* 42, pp. 93-114.

PUMA, A., “Due incisi sui cristiani nel *De pulsuum differentis* di Galeno e il suo preteso cristianesimo”, *PSM* 12.6, pp. 60-63.

RATHER, L.J., “The six things non-natural: a note on the origins and fate of a doctrine and frase”, *CM* 3 (1968) 337-347.

RIESE, W., "The structure of Galen's diagnostic reasoning", *Bull.N.Y.Acad.Med.* 44, pp. 778-791.

1967

ALLISON, F.G., "The life and times of Galen", *Manit.Med.Rev.* 46, pp. 635-637.

DURLING, R.J., "*Corringenda* and *addenda* to Diel's *Galenica*", *Traditio* 23, pp. 461-476.

EDELSTEIN, L., *Ancient Medicine*. Baltimore.

FORSSMAN, B., "ἐπὶ κάρ und ἀνὰ κάρ", *Glotta* 45, pp. 1-13.

JONES, C.P., "A friend of Galen", *CQ* 17, pp. 311-312.

KOLLESCH, J., "René Cartier, Herausgeber und Fäscher der Werke Galens", *Klio* 48, pp. 183-198.

MALATO, M.T., "Considerazioni nell'*Ars medicinalis Galenica* e sul commento Morgagnano", *Episteme* 1, pp. 81-86.

MANI, N., *Die Geschichte der Leherforschung von Galen bis Claude Bernard*. Basel.

SIEGEL, R.E., "Why Galen and Harvey did not compare the heart to a pump", *Am.J.Cardiol* 20, pp. 117-121.

STROHMAIER, G., "Hunayn ben Ishak al-Ibadi", in P. BEARMAN et al. (eds.), *Encyclopaedia of Islam*, pp. 578-581, Leiden.

1966

DE LACY, Ph., "Galen and the Greek poets", *GRBS* 7, pp. 259-266.

GOSS, C.M., "On anatomy of nerves by Galen of Pergamon", *Am.J.Anat* 118, pp. 327-335.

MALATO, M.T. and SCARANO, G.B., "Su di un esperimento di Galeno piu volte ripetuto e non ancora concluso", *Riv.Stor.Med* 10, pp. 194-205.

MARCOVICH, M., "Zu Aet. 5,23", *Hermes* 94, pp. 121-122.

McKEON, R., "Philosophy and the development of scientific methods", *JHI* 27, pp. 3-22.

MUNCH, I., "Antike Weltanschauung und Medizin II. Galen, Mediziner und Philosoph", *Hippokrates* 37, pp. 526-530.

O'MALLEY, C.D., "Galen (129-199 A.D.)", *Invest.Urol.* 3, pp. 427-428.

ONGARO, G., "La patologia epatica nel pensiero di Alessandro di Tralle", *Riv. di Storia dell. med.* 10, pp. 58-73.

PLESSNER, M., "Geschichte der Kinderheilkunde. Der Dresdner Pseudo-Galenus über Padagogik und Kinderhygiene", *Monatsschr. Kinderheilkd* 114, p. 479.

SCHUBRING, K., "Bibliographische Hingweise zu Galen", in C.G. Kühn (ed.), *Claudii Galeni Opera Omnia* Vol. XX, pp. XVII- LXII, Hildesheim.

STROHMAIER, G., "Eine bisher uberkannte Galen Schrift", *Helikon* 6, pp. 608-620.

TRIOLO, V.A., "An interpretative analysis of Galenic renal physiology", *CM* 1, pp. 113-128.

1965

GOSS, C.M., "The precision of Galen's anatomical descriptions compared with galenism". *Anat.Rec* 152, pp. 376-380.

KOLLESCH, J., "Aus Galens Praxis am römischen Kaiserhof", in E.C. WELSKOPF (ed.), *Neue Beiträge zur Geschichte der alten Welt II*, pp. 57–61, Berlin.

— "Galen und seine ärztliche Kollegen", *Altertum* 11, pp. 47-53.

LUTH, P., "Galen von Pergamon", *Med.Welt* 36, pp. 2072-2076.

LUTH, P. and KNAPP, W., "Der beste Arzt ist Wissenschaftler. Galen von Pergamon". *Med.Welt* 38, pp. 2185-2187.

RESCHER, N., "New light from Arabic sources on Galen and the fourth figure of the syllogism", *JHPh* 3, pp. 27-41.

STROHMAIER, G., "Galen als Vertreter der Gebildetenreligion seiner Zeit", *Neue Beitr. zur Gesch. der Alten Welt*, II, pp. 375-379.

VEITH, J., *Hystery: the history of a disease*. Chicago.

TABLE OF CONTENTS